Where
Did
Mary
Go?

Golden Age Series

The Adventure of Retirement:
It's About More Than Just Money
Guild A. Fetridge

After the Stroke: Coping with
America's Third Leading Cause
of Death
Evelyn Shirk

The Age of Aging: A Reader in
Social Gerontology
Abraham Monk

Between Home and Nursing Home:
The Board and Care Alternative
Ivy M. Down and Lorraine Schnurr

Caring for an Aging Parent:
Have I Done All I Can?
Avis Jane Ball

Caring for the Alzheimer Patient: A
Practical Guide, Second Edition
Raye Lynne Dippel, Ph.D., and
J. Thomas Hutton, M.D., Ph.D.

Caring for the Parkinson Patient:
A Practical Guide
J. Thomas Hutton, M.D., Ph.D., and
Raye Lynne Dippel, Ph.D.

Eldercare: Coping with
Late-Life Crisis
James Kenny, Ph.D., and
Stephen Spicer, M.D.

Geroethics: A New Vision of
Growing Old in America
Gerald A. Larue

Handle With Care: A Question
of Alzheimer's
Dorothy S. Brown

Long-Term Care in an Aging
Society: Choices and
Challenges for the '90s
Gerald A. Larue and Rich Bayly

My Parents Never Had Sex: Myths
and Facts of Sexual Aging
Doris B. Hammond, Ph.D.

On Our Own: Independent Living
for Older Persons
Ursula A. Falk, Ph.D.

Promises to Keep: The Family's Role
in Nursing Home Care
Katherine L. Karr

Taking Time for Me: How
Caregivers Can Effectively Deal
with Stress
Katherine L. Karr

Thy Will Be Done: A Guide to Wills,
Taxation, and Estate Planning
for Older Persons,
Revised Edition
Eugene J. Daley, Attorney at Law

Understanding "Senility":
A Layperson's Guide
Virginia Fraser and
Susan M. Thornton

When Blind Eyes Pierce the
Darkness: A Mother's Insights
Peter A. Angeles

When Living Alone Means Living at
Risk: A Guide for Caregivers
and Families
Robert W. Buckingham, Dr. P.H.

Working with the Elderly:
An Introduction
Elizabeth S. Deichman, Ed.M.,
ORT, and Regina Kociecki,
B.S.

You, Your Parent, and the
Nursing Home
Nancy Fox

Where Did Mary Go?

A Loving Husband's Struggle with Alzheimer's

FRANK A. WALL

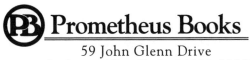 **Prometheus Books**

59 John Glenn Drive
Amherst, New York 14228-2197

Published 1996 by Prometheus Books

00 99 98 97 96   5 4 3 2 1

Library of Congress Cataloging-in-Publication Data

Wall, Frank A.
    Where did Mary go? / a loving husband's struggle with Alzheimer's / Frank A. Wall.
        p.   cm. — (Golden age series)
    ISBN 1–57392–070–3 (cloth : alk. paper)
    1. Wall, Mary M.—Health. 2. Alzheimer's disease—Patients—Family relationships. 3. Wall, Frank A. I. Title. II. Series.
RC523.2.W35W35   1996
362.1'96831'0092—dc20   96–16700
                                                          CIP

Printed in the United States of America on acid-free paper

Dedication

———➤•◄———

This book is dedicated to my wife, Mary, who struggled coura-
geously for several years against three overwhelming adversaries:
Parkinson's disease, Multi-infarct-dementia, and Alzheimer's disease; each in its own way systematically and progressively ravaged her mind and body. She lost her valiant struggle on July 19,
1992, when she succumbed to pulmonary asphyxiation.

This volume is also dedicated to thousands of unsung heroes,
the caregivers and other silent sufferers, who care at home for their
stricken loved ones. Too often they must watch in helpless disbelief while the minds and bodies of those for whom they care so
deeply pass beyond their ability to perform even the most basic
functions of everyday living to be swept away in a destructive current from which there is no escape.

Contents

———➤◆◄———

Foreword

I am honored to be asked to contribute a few comments to the book *Where Did Mary Go?* Over several years, I was a participant in and observer of the tragedy that Mary and Frank were the principal "players" in. They were both an inspiration to me throughout this long ordeal.

When I first met Mary, she was able to talk, though even then she was having to search for words at times. She appeared to have "pure" Parkinson's disease and initially responded positively to treatment with *carbidopa* (Sinemet®). I was cautiously optimistic but a little concerned about her speech difficulty. As time passed the situation became far more complex; Frank tells this story eloquently and graphically in this book.

I witnessed Mary's deterioration and Frank's courage evolve. As Mary's body and spirit crumbled, Frank's ability to cope grew and matured. Initially, she walked into my office with Frank. In time she came into my office with Frank holding her tightly against his body while she stood on his feet "walking." Then she

9

came in the wheelchair. I could recount other experiences and observations but will mention only one further.

Initially Mary could talk though there was a lack of fluency and some searching for words. This gradually deteriorated until she was finally mute. In her last months, her only "talking" was with her eyes, a condition which persisted, though to a very diminished degree, until a few months before her death. One intermediate stage will always be remembered by me. At one point, she could still sing with Frank. I shall never forget their rendition of "Let Me Call You Sweetheart" in my office at a time when she had lost all spontaneous speech. It was a truly memorable and highly emotional moment.

A remarkable fact about Frank is his ability to express himself candidly about subjects that are usually not discussed. I recall being a little surprised and taken aback by this candor in reading his *Mele Kalikimaka* (Hawaiian for "Merry Christmas") letter of 1991. People just don't discuss "poop and pee" so openly. I feel that one of the values of this book is this candor. Frank writes in a very matter-of-fact manner about things that are often considered embarrassing to discuss. He is also open about his feelings and reactions as he experienced them as Mary's caregiver during these trying years.

The greatest value of this book is Frank's willingness to share with the reader the day-to-day tasks that arise and the solutions that are discovered in dealing with a loved one with a dementing illness, regardless of the cause. In reading the manuscript, my confidence in the ability of a loving human as a caregiver to cope and innovate was again renewed. I think that those who are facing this formidable challenge will benefit from Frank's straightforward and sincere depiction of the life that he and Mary shared until her death. This book will help those caregivers stay on the "roller coaster" until the ride is finished.

James F. Pierce, M.D.
Honolulu, Hawaii

A Note from the Author

After years of caring for my wife, Mary, and reflecting on the many extraordinary experiences it entailed, numerous emotions, disbeliefs, and frustrations were triggered as each new emergency was confronted, as other significant challenges became everyday occurrences, and as the unexpected became the commonplace. In the hope of helping those who must now confront or who are awaiting the challenge of caregiving, I have highlighted some of the incidents which left a lasting impact on my memory:

- My utter disbelief at the doctor's early diagnosis. It was difficult to hear such bad news for Mary. At first I did not realize the real significance of what this illness could do. However, it did not take me long to learn this lesson. You always think you can beat the system, but in Mary's case it was not possible.
- The frequent frustrations I felt at not clearly understanding the destructive nature and fury of this terrible disease called de-

mentia. This term *dementia* meant nothing to me. It was just a medical term that applied to other people—not Mary or me. With the combined "terrible three"—Multi-infarct-dementia, Parkinson's disease, and Alzheimer's disease—I found out that it meant the end of all our dreams for retirement.

- Watching as its rapid progression along a destructive path stole the essential dignities of life from my loved one a piece at a time, right before my eyes.
- My uncertainty at the scope of this disease as it methodically reached into every corner of my wife's brain to destroy the mechanisms for control of her mental and physical capabilities.
- Coping with each new problem as it unfolded became part of a never-ending chain of tragic events that would remain forever deeply imprinted in my memories.
- The lessons I learned in dealing with life at its worst.
- My struggles to obtain even the smallest "respite" to save the part of my sanity which was slowly ebbing away.
- My early, fervent prayers that Mary would be healed, and later, my desperate pleas that she be spared the pain, suffering, and indignity.
- Finally I had to face the challenge of Mary's death, the grieving process, and then the need to get on with the rest of my life.

I gained a vast amount of knowledge through my firsthand experiences in all these areas and much more, all of which I will share with those of you who are taking on the challenge of caregiver. In retrospect, I wish I had such a volume to assist me when I took on my twenty-four-hour role as primary caregiver for my wife.

The task before you is awesome. It takes faith, knowledge, and courage, but above all *acceptance, patience,* and *love* to deal with the challenges you will encounter in the days, weeks, months, and, yes, years to come. For this difficult task you will need as much guidance as you can find.

Acknowledgments

I am deeply grateful to the many people who touched Mary's life and mine; they generously gave of their time, wisdom, and experience along with much-needed emotional support and encouragement during my lonely years as a caregiver and in researching and preparing the manuscript for this book. I thank you all.

To Mr. Carl Tapfer, caregiver for his wife (who is now deceased): you were my "wise counsel" in caregiving and you continue to be my close friend.

To my family, Robert, James, and Margaret, for their continuous close support for their mother and me during our long struggle.

To Dr. James F. Pierce, a top neurologist in Honolulu, who treated Mary with skill and friendship, and who provided me with personal understanding, medical advice, and a critical review of this book.

To Dr. James F. Wall, my son, for providing me with moral support and valuable medical information on care and treatment, and for his critical review of the manuscript for this book.

To Laurie Meininger, Executive Director of the Alzheimer's Association of Hawaii, for her professional expertise and constructive review of the manuscript of this volume.

To Karen Crozier, a public health nurse in Kaneohe, Hawaii, for her skill, kindness, and dedication to caring for those who so desperately need it. Also for her detailed review of this book.

And to all the various healthcare providers and facilities who cared for Mary over the years.

Prologue

———→•◦•←———

The doctors, scientists, and researchers still can't answer my nagging question: Where did Mary go?

After a very long and extremely stressful period of caring for Mary's every need twenty-four hours a day, every day of the year, I started to write as a way of "letting off steam" and to capture some of the many frustrations Mary and I were experiencing as her condition deteriorated. The writing was great therapy—I could get a lot off my chest—and at the same time, though I didn't appreciate it fully, I was recording my deepest feelings, which emerged while caregiving for Mary during the last seven years of her life. I would urge all caregivers to keep a journal and to make entries on a regular basis. Yes, you capture the anguish, guilt, and helplessness you feel all too often. But look deeper and you'll find precious memories and long-forgotten moments that you can cherish.

These words were prepared prior to Mary's sudden death on July 19, 1992.

Throughout the more than forty years we had been together

hard questions frequently confronted us, as with most marriages. Given enough time and sufficient information, most have been solved with logic and reason. But now I face my biggest question, one that defies all logic. And I must admit that it has me completely stumped. Where did Mary go?

Oh, her body is still here, though it's a shell of what used to be. The functions of life are barely noticeable as they continue to deteriorate at a rapid pace. The control mechanisms of Mary's mind and body have seriously malfunctioned; they are on a destructive course that is both progressive and irreparable. Mary's ability to recognize me or any of the people she once knew has fallen victim to dementia, which raises the companion question of "How much does Mary understand?" We just don't know. In this age of high technology we have eradicated many diseases, but medicine has yet to answer these nagging questions.

Sometimes a slight glimmer of recognition is clearly there, but it quickly vanishes into the unknown. How cruel this "dementia" is. I know she loves her daily shower, the head and body massages with the electric massager, riding in her wheelchair, and having her hair combed with soft strokes. Sometimes I see the satisfaction in her face or in her eyes.

New frustrations occur in direct correlation to the progressive nature of this terrible disease. In the past we eagerly looked forward to eating. Now each meal has become tedious and uncomfortable for both of us. Mary's inability to swallow and her constant coughing complicate an already difficult task. She needs her liquids for survival, but now it takes a syringe and a great deal of patience from both of us just to administer a drink of water or juice. Amen! She's finally taken some fluids. But the worst is yet to come: the big BM. In this regard normalcy is a thing of the past. Instead, a "digital procedure" is necessary. This takes courage, discipline, and a clothespin.

Where did Mary go? Actually, right now there are two Marys: the lovely, warm, and loving woman who resides in my memories and the woman trapped in the body and mind she now occupies. The doctors, scientists, and researchers don't know where my Mary went or why. Wherever she is, I hope she knows how very much she is loved.

Introduction

———➤◆◀———

This book is written for the many caregivers and families who struggle at home to serve the needs of loved ones with dementing illnesses. It is for those who have been (or will be) called upon, with or without prior notice or training, to perform the many complex and difficult tasks associated with one-on-one care of someone dear to them.

Information I will discuss comes from a vast storehouse of data compiled over many years of "hands-on" experience as the primary caregiver for my wife, Mary M. Wall. I will discuss in detail the tragic true story of her courageous seven-year struggle to survive in the unreal world of brain degeneration brought on by Multi-infarct-dementia (repeated small strokes), the neurological disorder known as Parkinson's disease, and the deteriorating brain disease known as Alzheimer's.

Each of these conditions is a formidable opponent, but Mary was a victim of all three—a deadly combination! Not one of these afflictions has a clear, identifiable cause or explanation. Certainly the doctors can pinpoint the physical source and the various likely factors that contributed to each disease occurring. But there seemed to be nothing Mary or I could have done to stop them from invading her body and mind. There are no positive cures with ready-made over-the-counter remedies that hold the promise of restoring the normal basic functions of everyday living. Victims like Mary and the loved ones who share their lives can only stand by helplessly as vital human functions are tragically and dramatically stolen in a ruthless and insidiously progressive way by these various forms of dementia.

As Mary's primary caregiver over the years, I was an eyewitness to her one-way journey along a highly emotional road toward an all too predictable destination. The road was treacherous, with serious obstacles at every turn and with many tragic accidents en route.

Nothing in my military background or in my business experience could have prepared me for the unbelievable challenges I lived through during those years. There were many things to learn but so little time to grasp them. Of necessity I had to perform a variety of caregiving functions that I was ill-prepared to assume and I found myself having to make decisions on a great many levels, some involving life-and-death situations.

Through countless discussions with doctors, nurses, technicians, other caregivers, and support groups; courses and seminars, books, articles, and library research; along with the hard work of "learning by doing," I grew into my new role as a caregiver. It wasn't easy, but I had a compelling incentive to learn quickly. A human life was depending on me *every day* for *everything*.

At first I actually believed I could take care of Mary by myself. As the disease rapidly progressed with new problems mounting daily, I realized this was an impossible dream. The toll on me was too great. I needed help or at least some respite time so that I could properly carry out my prime responsibilities of caring for Mary. Toward this end I targeted day-care facilities for respite, often difficult to get in due to shortages and long waiting lists. I was able to bring Mary to several facilities over the course of her illness for short periods during the day, usually for a few hours. Most of the respite time was used for essential errands, shopping for groceries, picking up medical supplies and prescriptions, going to my doctor's appointments, and other non-fun activities. Yes, I would take respite any way I could get it—within reason. The remainder of the time I was there for Mary. The prime responsibility for her care and life was mine. I discuss this matter in various chapters throughout the book. Remember that respite is as important for you as care is for your stricken loved one.

Mary is gone now and my caregiving days have come to an end. I could just file away all these years of hands-on experience and move on to more pleasant pursuits. But then I'll hear of someone else who just learned that their loved one faces a debilitating, possibly terminal disease that will require their dedicated efforts as a caregiver. At that point I feel compelled to pass on my hard- earned experience to those who will follow me in their new roles as caregivers.

In the pages that follow I will describe as frankly and as clearly as I can the many facets of caregiving: the problems, frustrations, and emotions patients and caregivers confront; some tips, suggestions, and even a solution or two when faced with what seems to be an insurmountable set of problems; and a roadmap of what to expect as the disease progresses in your loved one. Specifically I will address the following:

- The illnesses: Multi-infarct-dementia, Parkinson's disease, and Alzheimer's disease.
- Information on various medical aids to assist in the caregiving function and identification of some important medical terms to enhance understanding of the disease and its treatment.
- Contrasting "the way life used to be" for Mary and me during happier times in an atmosphere of family love and laughter, with the chilling effects of this disease on her mind and body.

- Some of the signals, symptoms, and reactions that portend future unknown problems such as mental confusion, incontinence, falling, wandering, and related concerns.
- Recognition that "something is really wrong"; trying to pin down, understand, and gain a fix on the ongoing devastating problems caused by the disease.
- Confronting "the hard facts of life" and how these facts affect the patient, the caregiver, and the family. Accepting the reality of Mary's disease.
- Feeding someone who has problems swallowing. Preparing the foods and liquids, developing a nutritious diet, and the value of food supplements.
- The chronology of Mary's mental and physical deterioration as the disease progressed, and a pictorial look at some of the actual details of the rapid physical decline of her body.
- Mary's reaction to the decline of her mind and body, and her ability (or inability) to cope with her disease. How the disease affected me and the rest of the family. The many sacrifices that were made in a valiant but unsuccessful effort to restore the way things used to be.
- The dilemma of the "inexperienced caregiver" suddenly pressed into service under stress and emotion to care for a loved one in all facets of everyday living. In addition, I'll offer a detailed discussion of caring for the caregiver.
- The signs and changes that indicate a transition to the terminal period. I'll discuss how the end came, detailing the tragic events that resulted in Mary's death. After which the caregiver must deal with shock, planning the burial, and getting all the person's affairs in order. I'll explain the grieving process and how to get on with the rest of your life.
- Some of the many practical lessons I learned over the years, presented in a format that can provide new caregivers insights on what to expect and how to cope with some of the trials and tragedies of caring for your patient.

- This discussion will assist other caregivers of those affected by dementia, increase their understanding of these problems and solutions, help them avoid some of the pitfalls associated with care in the home, and provide a roadmap of what to expect as the disease progresses.

1

About the Disease

DEMENTIA

The word *dementia* comes from the Latin words "away" and "mind." Doctors define it as a loss or impairment of mental powers. Dementia describes a group of symptoms, but it is not a disease. The symptoms include, among others: mental confusion, memory loss, disorientation, and intellectual impairment. The concept of dementia incorporates several diseases, among them Alzheimer's disease, Multi-infarct-dementia, and Parkinson's disease. Each has a direct correlation to the loss or impairment of mental control of certain brain functions resulting in the retardation or elimination of the victim's ability to perform basic functions of everyday living. Each is progressive and irreparable and all eventually end in death.

My Mary was a victim of all of these diseases—a deadly combination. The doctors did not have a plausible answer to the question, "Why did Mary have all three of these diseases at the same time?"

Alzheimer's Disease

Alzheimer's disease is a progressive, irreversible, and fatal brain disease recognized as one of the most devastating maladies of our time. As the fourth leading cause of death among adults in the United States, it is responsible for more than one hundred thousand deaths annually. The symptoms include gradual memory loss, disorientation, impaired personality changes, and finally loss of control over body functions. Its victims are eventually rendered incapable of caring for themselves. Brain activity gradually diminishes until the patient lapses into a coma and dies. The cause of the illness is not known, and there is no known cure or medication to stop its progress. There are various drugs that claim to slow the brain deterioration, but these must often be taken very early on. While researchers continue seeking causes and cures, much has been done to diminish the patient's behavioral and emotional symptoms.

The latest advance in the treatment of dementia of the Alzheimer's type is a new drug called Cognex (also known as tetrahydroaminoacridine, tracine, or THA). This drug, approved by the U.S. Food and Drug Administration in September 1993, is the first medication developed specifically to treat Alzheimer's disease. Though not a cure, the hope is that it can slow the progression of the disease. In clinical studies Cognex has provided some benefits for Alzheimer's patients in the early stages of the disease. This medication is now available by prescription from your doctor. It is very important to have a thorough discussion with your physician about the possible benefits, risks, and costs in order to decide whether or not to try this drug.

Alzheimer's disease is not a natural part of aging; people in their fifties and sixties as well as those much older have been diagnosed. Nor is the disease easily diagnosed. Treatment or care of patients with Alzheimer's is not covered by government or most private insurance.

In 1984 Mary began showing some of the symptoms of

Alzheimer's disease. After she was admitted to Castle Medical Center in Kailua, these symptoms led a supervising doctor to suspect Mary had Alzheimer's. During observations and examinations the doctors periodically noted touches of memory loss, confusion, impaired judgment, personality changes, and some loss of language skills in varying degrees. Although she continued to have these symptoms to a greater degree in the later stages of her illness, positive confirmation of Mary having Alzheimer's disease must come from a postmortem. This was confirmed by the official autopsy performed on Mary after her death.

This disease is an emotional and financial nightmare for both the victims and their families. The economic impact of the disease is staggering with the estimated cost of care reaching as high as $90 billion dollars annually and growing. Over four million Americans are afflicted: one in ten over age sixty-five, according to the Alzheimer's Association Research Organization.

Multi-infarct-dementia

This disease is also called *Vascular Dementia,* caused by repeated strokes which destroy small areas of the brain. The cumulative effect of this damage leads to dementia. Multi-infarct-dementia affects several brain functions including memory, coordination, or speech, depending on what part of the brain was damaged. It normally progresses in a steplike manner. Often the strokes that occur are unperceptible; there are no outward signs like paralysis or slurred speech.

Stroke is a form of cardiovascular disease. It affects the arteries and veins of the brain and stops the flow of blood bringing oxygen and nutrients. A stroke can occur when one or more of these blood vessels either burst, thereby flooding an area of the brain with blood and cutting off its oxygen, or become clogged with a blood clot, in which case it starves the affected area. Part of the brain doesn't receive the flow of blood it needs because of the rupture or blockage; as a result it starts to die.

The key warning signals of a stroke, according to the researchers of the American Heart Association, are:

- Sudden weakness or numbness of the arm and leg on one side of the body;
- Loss of speech or trouble talking or understanding speech;
- Dimness or loss of vision, particularly in one eye;
- Unexplained dizziness (especially when associated with other neurologic symptoms);
- Unsteadiness or falls;
- Sudden severe headaches with no apparent cause.

Some multi-infarct-dementias can be stopped by preventing further strokes. In others progression of the disease cannot be stopped.

Parkinson's Disease

According to the United Parkinson Foundation, *Parkinson's* is a progressive disease of the nervous system characterized by involuntary tremors, rigidity of muscles, and slowness of movement. The disease involves a deficiency of the chemical *dopamine* in the brain. With this deficiency there is a loss of smooth, rapid movement of the limbs. It occurs most commonly in the aged, though here, too, the disease has been known to affect much younger people.

Parkinson's disease does not actually diminish a person's mental faculties, although these may appear to be impaired once the victim's speech is affected.

The cause of this disease is often not known. It is thought to be caused by arteriosclerosis (hardening of the arteries), in which there is degeneration of the brain cells that control body movements. Parkinsonism also may be caused by a brain tumor, brain damage, or from chemicals such as manganese and carbon dioxide. There is as yet no known cure, but the symptoms can be controlled in early stages by drug treatment with *levodopa* (L-dopa [Sinemet®]).

The later stages of Parkinson's disease may include continuous hand tremors, pill rolling (continually moving the fingers forward on one or both hands in a circular motion), arms held in a bent position, and the body bent forward in permanent stoop. The patient may also walk slowly with shuffling steps and then start to run forward. This is called *festination walk.* Parkinson's victims may have handwriting that is small and illegible, and their speech may become slurred or unintelligible.

Research continues on each of these disease areas, but at this writing no positive cures have been developed.

2

The Way Things Used to Be

⫸•⫷

Mary and her sister, Margaret, were identical twins, and quite beautiful, not only in the eyes of those who loved them, but also in the eyes of the community of Santa Barbara, California, which selected the twins to ride in the seat of honor on the "Santa Barbara Float" entered in the 1936 Rose Bowl Parade in Pasadena. How happy and proud they were to be representing their town before the whole world.

Mary was an energetic and petite woman with naturally wavy brunette hair, beautiful facial features and body contours, and silky smooth skin. She always wore a friendly smile. People turned for a second look as she passed them.

It was 1939, when the twins were living in San Francisco, that I came into Mary's life. A friend of mine was seeing Mary and he invited me to join them on a double date. I reluctantly went along only as a favor to my friend. But from the moment Mary and I met, a fire was lighted between us that was to remain forever. Of course my friend was hurt, but he remained close to Mary and me for many years.

During our early courtship Mary and her sister planned a party. I was a civilian student pilot and my college buddy had just graduated from the U.S. Army "Flying Cadet Program" at Randolph Field, Texas. I mentioned this to Mary, who replied, "Yes, invite your buddy and his two friends to come to the party." They had just been transferred to Hamilton Field, California, across the bay from Mary's apartment.

The night of the party many people attended. All of a sudden three brand-new convertible cars screeched to a halt in front of Mary's apartment, and three newly commissioned Army Air Force second lieutenants wearing their newly won wings and distinctive uniforms climbed out. They had just graduated from a tough grind and were ready to howl. I must be nuts inviting these "top guns" to steal my girl!

Sure enough, upon their arrival my friend zeroed in on Mary. It wasn't long before he had her cornered. I immediately came to her rescue (and mine) by politely grabbing his arm and saying, "This is my girl. In the next room there's one just like her. You can have her."

The same fire that ignited me caught him as well. It was love at first sight. The two married before Mary and I did. Now I have a dear friend who has been my brother-in-law for years and remains one of my very best friends.

I well remember my days as a second lieutenant when Mary and I were often invited to dine at the colonel's table at the Officers' Club. I thought I must have been doing something very right to receive such an honor. Actually, it was Mary's stunning good looks.

It was hard to tell Mary and her sister apart. They were interchangeable in appearance, but I could always tell who was who. One day, Mary decided to take the day off from work. So she asked Margaret, who wasn't working that day, to take her place as a hatcheck girl at the Sir Francis Drake Hotel in San Francisco. Margaret was briefed on details of the job and then reported for duty. No one could tell that a deception had taken place. It was hard to believe.

As I think back, so much has changed from the way things used to be. When I first met Mary she was a beautiful accomplished ballroom dancer who was contemplating a career as a professional dancer—that is until we met and her plans were changed forever. We loved to dance and did often until her illness made it impossible.

While I was on unaccompanied military assignments Mary was the head of the house, becoming mother and father to our three small children, Robert, James, and Margaret. She made the necessary decisions. She cared for the children when they were sick. She took them to doctor's appointments, to school functions, to the playing field, and much more. Mary was a fabulous mother and wife. There was no problem she couldn't solve.

Mary was a companion and helper. She was always pitching in to do more than her share of the work to create a home atmosphere each time we moved—and we moved quite often: Alabama, New Mexico, Texas, Virginia, Florida, California, Illinois, Missouri, Oklahoma, Guam, Japan, and Hawaii, to name a few of our stations. It was difficult for the whole family to pull up roots and move to a new location with all the attendant packing, transportation arrangements, pacifying of the kids, finding new schools, leaving old friends and meeting new ones, all the while moving with mixed feelings of sadness and anticipation. Mary was always there with a helping hand and in the middle of everything.

When I retired from active service in the air force in February 1977, Mary and I would eagerly plan our trips to many places around the world. It was stimulating, interesting, and fun. The frenzy of arranging transportation and travel itineraries, overseeing the packing, and finally getting on the aircraft to zoom into the sky on a new adventure was great fun for both of us. How I miss those trips together.

It was fun when all the children, now with kids of their own, would occasionally congregate at home in Hawaii away from their homes strewn across the country and overseas. We had a hilarious time, with much confusion as everyone would update everyone else on all the news since they had last met. Mary was in the thick of everything then, but the last few years she became subdued and withdrawn, shying away from even talking to family members as if in a world of her own with no real recognition of her family or desire to be with her loved ones.

Mary was my friend and confidante for forty-nine years. When she listened to my problems they would just melt away, solved through love and understanding. My usual greeting of "Hey, honey, I'm home" has no meaning now that I'm alone. The house is being renovated, but something big is missing and it will be hard to replace. The gaiety and laughter has been supplanted with emptiness. There's no one to greet me, to prepare my meals, to share my confidences.

For seven years I was eyewitness to Mary's involuntary and grotesque transformation from a vibrant, robust woman to a ravaged old lady unable to perform normal functions, to talk, or even to let me know how she was coping with this onslaught of brain degeneration. It remains a mystery to this day.

I condensed some of my feelings and observations in a 1990 Christmas letter to our many friends and family:

"ALOHA" and "MELE KALIKIMAKA"—1990

This was a year of remembering—how it "was" and how it "is now."

Mary again is the subject. She remains totally dependent on me for everything. I mean everything! The only things she can do with ease and without her knowledge is "pee and poop." Sometimes pee only, sometimes poop only, sometimes pee and poop, but it's there every day of the year. During the past three years—going on thirty—I've changed enough "diapers" to pave the way to the moon.

Things were not always that way. I remember:

How meticulous she was in her dress and grooming. She was the most beautiful Colonel's Lady—so graceful and pretty. Today she wears diapers and dusters, but she still looks like a queen.

How vivacious she was with her gaiety and laughter; everyone watched as we so skillfully skimmed over the dance floor. Waltzes were her favorite. Today, when I play some of the old waltzes a glimmer of remembrance glistens in her eye as she tries to "sing along" but can't.

When we would go on long walks through the fantastically beautiful landscape of mountains, oceans, and hills here in Hawaii. How eagerly she looked forward to those daily walks. But today it's a ride in the wheelchair in a horizontal position with a quizzical look into the sky as if in another world. She is in another world most of the time.

The frenzied pace and the last-minute packing when we would go on our many trips to see friends and visit places all over the world. In retrospect, while at times it was a bit frustrating, it was also very stimulating and fun. Today our travel is limited to the doctor, the hospital, the clinic, and the pharmacy. Preparation for these trips is also frustrating: changing her, dressing her, getting the diaper bag ready, getting into and out of the car, stowing the wheelchair in the car, etc. Planning is a must every step of the way. Spontaneity is normally not an option.

The wonderful homecooked meals Mary prepared over the years. What a cook—or should I say "Super Chef." How I miss her in "Mother's Kitchen" preparing the family meals. Talking about it makes me hungry. Today this role is reversed. I must do all these chores. She is a tough act to follow. She never complains about my cooking; of course, she can't talk. I now understand why Mary would often say, "Lets eat out tonight." I still take her to a restaurant once a week. It's very difficult. The stares of those unknown to you have changed from admiration of a beautiful woman to what appears to be those of "sympathy" or "caring," but I'll do it until I am unable to handle her or to cope!

One always assumes catastrophic illnesses only happen to "other people." Don't you believe it. It could happen to YOU!

I have earned many degrees, awards, citations, and certificates over the years, but the one I received this month means more to me than all the rest. It was a certificate for being a family caregiver. It was one truly earned through love; patience; and a lot of blood, sweat, and tears.

I knew it; I'm going to run out of space. So let's get right to the Christmas message for 1990. Do your living today because tomorrow may never come. Take care of your health *before* it's too late. Take care of each other because no one else will. God bless you all—Have a wonderful holiday and 1991.

Till we meet again in 1991.

MARY   ANDY/FRANK

(From the Walls)

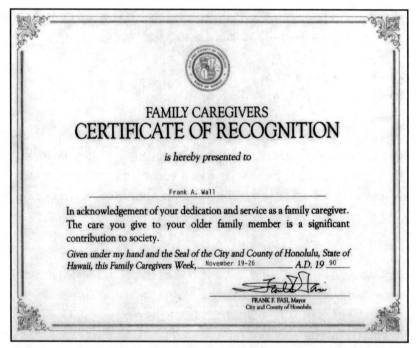

Certificate of Recognition awarded to Frank A. Wall during Family Caregivers Week, November 19–26, 1990. The Elderly Affairs Division, County of Honolulu, honored family caregivers while informing the community on the importance of caregiver services and the need to support their efforts.

3

Something Is Wrong with Mary

Several symptoms of change in Mary's behavior began to occur in late 1984 when she was sixty-four, but I mistakenly considered them "nothing to worry about." For example, Mary was a highly efficient keeper of the bankbook. In the past she would breeze through the balancing process with skill, speed, and accuracy. Then she started to have extreme difficulty in performing even the *simplest calculations*. She would end up saying in very frustrated tones, "I can't do it! I can't do it! I just can't do it!"

This performance was a clear signal that a small but significant change was taking place in Mary's mental control system. It didn't last and I dismissed it in my mind as nothing serious, not knowing the present or future ramifications of this seemingly isolated event. Nor did I try to find out what was happening to my wife. This was my first clue.

Later that year Mary started to have some *mental confusion* and a distinct memory deficit on a short-term basis. For example, she would ask me to explain how to push the control buttons on the TV remote control device. I clearly explained this simple operation in painstaking detail. Minutes later she would track me down and repeatedly ask me: "How does this thing work? I can't do it!" She would repeat this after each explanation given to her. In hindsight, this was another clear signal that, however small, a dementia problem existed which was not acted on.

In early 1985 Mary's *posture* became somewhat unnatural. She was bending slightly forward. Another symptom which was brushed aside.

We continued to play golf, go on trips, attend the theater, and go to football games. At last, we were starting to enjoy our retired life in this Hawaiian paradise. In mid-1985, while she was attempting to putt the golf ball into a hole on the green, Mary suddenly *fell* on her face onto the green. She looked at me quizzically and said, "It's nothing, let's continue to play." This was the alarm that spurred me to action.

As we continued to play golf, the frequency of her falls was slowly but methodically increasing and expanding to other areas. The golf staff marveled at her guts and courage to continue with the game. But Mary was like that. In just a few months, she could no longer hit the ball, but would carry a golf club and swing it aimlessly into the air as she accompanied me on a round of golf at the Hickam Air Force Base Par-3 golf course. It was a type of therapy for her.

The next noticeable symptom was Mary's difficulty in getting up or out of a chair once she was seated. She would struggle several times before eventually getting herself into a standing position. In time this problem became progressively worse. Then came the *festination walk*—a tendency to walk in short fast steps while bending forward, all the while with a sensation of falling forward. If this weren't enough, Mary also suffered from *rigidity.* Her arms would be very tightly pressed to her body with extreme tenseness. Often I had to pry her arms from her side. These were some of the early symptoms that occurred in a methodical manner over a period of several months.

Mary's condition was diagnosed as Parkinson's disease by Dr. James F. Pierce, a top neurologist in Honolulu. He reached this conclusion based upon the symptoms Mary presented and after exhaustive tests and examinations. Dr. Pierce immediately gave her a prescription for Sinemet®, a drug to replenish the chemical dopamine which the brain needed but could no longer manufacture due to the deterioration of a section of its tissue.

Almost overnight Mary responded to this medication. At this early stage I called it the miracle drug. Once again I had my lovely Mary back. She could do all those functions which before taking the medication she could not do: getting up, flexibility, proper walking gait, straight posture, and recovered balance. I thought to myself, Parkinson's disease is a piece of cake; we can live with this and we did. But the honeymoon of Mary's return to normalcy was short-lived.

At this point we thought we had a positive identification of Mary's problem, and we were right—but only in part.

After discussing these incidents with Dr. Pierce, he said there is something unusual going on in Mary's brain and we must get to the bottom of it. He ordered an MRI scan (Magnetic Resonance Imagery) of Mary's brain. The CT scans previously taken did not identify any stroke problems. The CT scanner is a machine that passes X rays through the patient's body from various angles, which enables a computer to build up three-dimensional images to pinpoint problems. It can concentrate on a specific area of the body such as the brain. This was done in Mary's case. Results of the MRI scan revealed that Mary had suffered several minor strokes. Now we were given yet another part of the puzzle— Multi-infarct-dementia (minor strokes), Parkinson's disease, and possibly Alzheimer's disease.

The diagnosis suggested *possible* Alzheimer's disease because the disease can be positively identified only after death in a post-mortem. When I received the doctor's diagnosis, inwardly I felt devastated. I discussed it with Mary; however, I don't believe she could comprehend the severity of the disease or its impact on her future.

Mary faced a triple threat; each was progressive and irreparable. It was now confirmed that something was actually wrong with Mary. With this new knowledge we were better able to deal with the current problems and to be somewhat aware of new ones that might occur in the future. Mary was now well on her journey down the destructive path to hardship, pain, and mental and physical deterioration.

Looking back, many incidents occurred that revealed additional signs directly pointing to dementia, a deterioration of brain cells resulting in the malfunction of the ability of mind and body to function normally.

The body can give many signals of a dementia problem that portends big trouble in the future. In the early stages they are normally insignificant and can easily be overlooked as nothing to worry about. When they occur on a frequent or infrequent basis it is important for you to seek medical evaluation and diagnosis. Many times early detection and positive identification of the problem is possible. In Mary's case, the series of events that occurred in the early stages of her disease should have alerted me to take early medical action, but they were not acted on. Signals from the body are seldom wrong and should be acted upon.

The caregiver, in coordination with family members when possible, must work out guilt feelings. A key factor in this regard is if you feel you could have actually changed anything. In Mary's situation very little could have been changed.

What follows is a quick recap of the progression of Mary's deterioration over the years, up to the time of her death in July 1992, including the "milestone events" that resulted in Mary's inability to perform the basic functions of everyday living:

1. Difficulty in performing minor calculations

2. Inability to drive her car

3. Short-term mental deficits

4. Confusion

5. An inability to get up once seated

6. Rigidity in the arms and holding them close to the body

7. Unnatural posture—bending over and forward

8. Festination walk—the sensation of falling forward

9. Inability to participate intelligently in "verbal conversation"

10. Incontinence of the bladder—uncontrolled release of urine

11. Loss of ability to use the toilet

12. Loss of ability to talk

13. Erratic behavior—getting up at 3 A.M. to cook dinner

14. Uncontrolled falls

15. Inability to dress herself

16. Inability to shower and care for her personal hygiene

17. Inability to groom herself

18. Susceptibility to urinary tract infection

19. Inability to eat without assistance

20. Inability to walk

21. Incontinence of bowel—uncontrolled bowel movement

22. Right leg contracting—becoming stiff and extended

23. Right hand curling into a tight fist

24. Excessive loss of weight

25. Choking on food, water, and saliva

26. Need for a suction machine to clear the throat of phlegm, mucus, etc.

27. Need for pureed food and food supplements

28. Bedsores and decubitus ulcers on sides and back

29. Both hands and wrists curling tightly with fingernails digging deeply into flesh

30. Becoming the classic "basket case." Near the end Mary was unable to perform any normal body function. Her right leg was contracted, her hands curled inward, and at times she appeared to be returning to her fetal position.

The final event came when aspiration of food into the lungs, choking, and the cutting off of oxygen to the brain resulted in heart failure and death.

4

A Chronology of Symptoms, Problems, and Happenings

In late 1984 Mary and I went on an extended visit to California. During the trip she became withdrawn. When visiting her sister Margaret she did not enter into discussions with her—very unusual for Mary. When I talked with her she was unable to comprehend what was said. She was also being treated for depression. Upon our return Mary was admitted to Castle Medical Center in Kailua for testing and observation. A supervising doctor diagnosed Mary as having a short-term memory deficit and suspected she had Alzheimer's disease. This was the first indication that she had a dementia problem.

Mary and I discussed this problem in some detail and were shocked at the diagnosis. Neither of us had any idea what the disease was except that it affects other people. This was the beginning of my education on Alzheimer's and dementia-related diseases. In retrospect Mary showed no real reaction to what was happening or what was in store for her other than to shake it off as nothing to worry about.

Each of the three diseases attacked Mary *incrementally*: first Alzheimer's, then Parkinson's, and finally Multi-infarct-dementia. I was coping with the first one and trying to get a handle on it when the next one would come up. There always seemed to be another problem just ahead. Identification of Parkinson's and minor strokes was possible; however, the only positive way of identifying Alzheimer's is by autopsying the deceased. The autopsy performed on Mary by the medical examiners after her death confirmed that she had in fact been suffering from Alzheimer's disease. The actual details of each of these attacks on Mary are discussed in the appropriate chapters of this book.

Dr. James F. Pierce, a top neurologist in Honolulu, diagnosed Mary as having Parkinson's disease, Multi-infarct-dementia, and possibly Alzheimer's disease after many examinations and tests including MRI scans. He confirmed that Mary's early symptoms were Parkinson's. The MRI scans he ordered showed Mary had suffered several minor strokes and the autopsy confirmed Alzheimer's.

News of the diagnosis was devastating to our family. Many things flashed through my mind. Is this what the golden years of retirement are all about? This is not fair to Mary! How am I going to handle this problem? Mary appeared aloof to the problem. All the children were very concerned about their mother, but due to distance were able to visit infrequently, and communicated their feelings through phone calls, letters, and flowers, which were appreciated very much by Mary and me.

The following chronology details what happened to Mary during her struggle with the three diseases of dementia.

During the perilous journey on the "dementia path" you can expect many unusual situations to arise. Some will be bizarre, interesting, or even humorous, while others could be tragic, sad, or devastating. Those I can recall—the ones that left unforgettable impressions on my mind—are identified in what follows. In your role as a caregiver, any of these events could happen to your loved one.

FALLING

In early 1985, I had to leave the house for an important appointment. I advised Mary not to leave the house. At this point she could talk a little and had some understanding. When I returned at 3 P.M. Mary was gone. Where had she gone? I looked everywhere including our favorite walking routes. I contacted the neighbors and then went through the streets of the neighborhood searching for her. It was now getting late and still no clue of where Mary could be.

I called the police at 6 P.M. and filed a missing person report but continued the search to no avail. Then came the rains. It was coming down in torrents. I was getting frantic. It was now 8 P.M. with a cloudburst continuing in the area. The whole neighborhood was searching in different places, but still no Mary.

Then came the first clue: a neighbor had been in the Haiku Garden Restaurant across the street from our house. The manager had verified to a neighbor that someone answering to Mary's description had eaten there, but could not sign the check (she was unable to write). I immediately talked to the manager, who recalled seeing Mary go down into the beautiful tropical gardens by way of their "garden walk," a long winding path into the dense gardens of Haiku. But no one saw her return.

One neighbor had traversed the path for a short distance and had not seen Mary. I was advised of this on my telephone answering machine. It was now established that Mary had in fact been there.

I retraced the path into the tropical forest. As I approached the very end, a member of the search party called out, "Frank, you'd better get over here quick." It was now 9 P.M.

It was very dark, and raining so hard you could not see your hands in front of you. Then I glanced at Mary. She was on the ground in a prone position with her head sloping down toward a large tree trunk. She was being pelted mercilessly by the hard rain. She couldn't move. Her eyes were open but with a glazed, unknowing stare. She was cold and clammy with a low pulse. I bundled her up and carried her back through the long, dark, wet path to our house. There I dried and changed her, put blankets on her, and gave her hot drinks. Once she was warm and dry, we were off to the hospital emergency room at Tripler Army Medical Center. The examining doctor said that Mary's six-hour stay on the wet ground had miraculously caused no serious injury. But had I not gone to the very end of the path she probably would not have survived the night. *God was surely by her side that night.* After nine hours she was finally safely tucked into her bed for the night. What an experience!

This was just her first fall. It was followed by many others with far more serious consequences.

One day, while in our family room, I heard a loud cracking thump. It sounded like something crashing against the wall. I ran into the bedroom to find Mary on the floor of the walk-in closet with an odd cheshire-cat grin on her face. I also found a gaping hole in the wall of the closet where her head had struck it.

She had attempted to put on her skirt, but lost her balance and fell hard, hitting her head against the wallboard and breaking right through. What a hit, and this was only the beginning.

Another scene was played out while we were sitting in the family room watching TV. Although she couldn't understand it she seemed to be intrigued by the movement on the screen. All of a sudden she bolted up from her seat and immediately lost her balance and fell hard backward into the jalousie windows, breaking two glass panes and sustaining a severe cut on the back of her head requiring another trip to the emergency room and a number of stitches.

Yet another episode occurred when I took her with me to the bank. She was fastened in her seatbelt with the car door locked and I felt sure she was secure. I was just being waited on by the teller when I glanced to my right and in a flash I saw Mary walking toward me. In that brief moment she had taken a hard fall on her back and head causing a loud cracking noise. I ran to her side and took her home after a cursory inspection of her head. You guessed it—another trip to the emergency room, where the X rays revealed no problems.

Mary's falls were becoming a habit. After the incident at the bank two more falls in the bedroom resulted in severe bumps on her head and deep impressions on the wallboards.

Despite my best efforts, Mary would no longer sit quietly. She was continually trying to get up, only to fall again. She did this several times one day. I would leave the room for barely a minute or I might even be in the same room and that all too familiar bump would sound and Mary would be on the floor. At this point I just couldn't control her falling. Mary's safest place seemed to be on the floor.

After several falls I took her to Tripler Medical Center where she was admitted for observation. She remained there for three weeks during which time many tests were taken. It also gave me a much-needed respite.

One recommendation from the hospital was to put Mary in a wheelchair and secure her with a *posey restraint,* a tie-in-jacket put on like a sweater with strings that are attached to the wheelchair to secure her. I had mixed feelings about using the restraint. I didn't like tying her down, but it was the safest thing to do and would provide me some assurance she would not be falling. I took the advice and acquired the restraint.

Soon thereafter I had Mary secured in the wheelchair and for the first time in quite a while I really began to feel *safe* when I went out of the room. It was the morning after I picked up Mary from the hospital. I had gone into the shower confident that Mary was safe. I had just soaped up in the shower when I heard a loud crashing sound followed by a blood-chilling scream. My God! What had happened?

I dashed to the family room to find Mary all tangled up in the overturned wheelchair. Blood streaming from her forehead was dripping onto the wheelchair and the newly shampooed rug. So this is what they call security!

The problem was simple enough and I was able to fix it so future crashes couldn't occur. I looped the straps of the restraint over the wheelchair handles. This secured Mary, making it impossible for her to stand up in the wheelchair.

Not surprisingly, the wheelchair incident resulted in yet another trip to the emergency room (the staff there knew us on sight). Several new stitches were needed to close the wound. Mary's scars were mounting!

The wheelchair now became the prime means of moving Mary from one place to another. Even though she was technically ambulatory, securing her to the wheelchair made her life safer and mine a lot less frazzled.

After these injuries I had no choice but to use the posey restraint. I also used it to secure her in her seat in the family room and at night in her bed. Yes, it sounds like jail, and no doubt it was very confining to her, but the restraint was used only for her own safety. I agonized over it, but in the end using the restraint was the right thing to do.

At this early stage of her illness she was not safe even with skilled caregivers. She had an insatiable desire to continually get up, whether she was located in a chair, in bed, or in her wheelchair. At times it seemed she was rebelling against the diseases that were taking away her normal functions bit by bit.

During her "falling period" Mary's actions reminded me of a "punch drunk" boxer who, after being knocked down by his opponent, would get up again, only to be knocked down once more. She was a very gutsy lady. It was an extremely sad episode in Mary's tragic experience with dementia.

UNPREDICTABLE BEHAVIOR

Very early one morning (4 A.M. to be exact) I found Mary unloading the dishwasher. I was in bed and thought she was, too. This time I was awakened by a tremendous crashing sound. I found Mary on the kitchen floor under a pile of seven broken dinner plates. I asked what happened, but of course she couldn't explain. It was clear to me that she overestimated her capacity to lift that many at one time and then tried to lift them into the second tier shelf in the kitchen cabinet. She lost her balance and fell. This occurred in the early stages of her disease.

At 3 A.M. I heard a noise coming from the kitchen, along with an unusual aroma permeating the master bedroom. I turned over in bed to check Mary, but she was not there. I dashed into the kitchen to see a pathetic display of *confusion.* All the burners on the stove were on high, while dishes, plates, and pans were scattered all over the kitchen counters. Food was on the counters and the floor. I said, "Why are you doing this at 3 A.M.?" She smiled at me and said, "I'll have dinner in a few minutes." Her internal time clock and coordinating capability were malfunctioning. She used to start getting things ready for dinner around 4 P.M.

It was Christmas holidays (1989) and two of our three children were home. A part-time caregiver was handling Mary. The caregiver and Mary were walking down the hallway with Mary on the left as they approached the open bathroom door, which is also on the left. Mary jerked her arm away from the caregiver and in one split second she had taken another hard fall onto the tiled bathroom floor. This time Mary was silent. She had long since lost her ability to scream.

My son Jim, a doctor, who was visiting us, immediately treated her, but it still resulted in another trip to the hospital emergency room. This time several stitches on her forehead were required.

Another episode occurred about 2 A.M. I was awakened by the slamming of a door. I jumped out of bed in search of Mary. I found her in the kitchen with a half-gallon container of chocolate ice cream (her favorite) on the counter. With ice cream smeared all over her face, hair, nightgown, and body, she was digging with her hands into the container and scooping it out with her right hand and wiping her ice-cream-covered left hand on her nightgown. Ice cream was all over the floor. I had quite a time trying to get her to stop digging into the ice cream. She seemed to be protecting it from me. She had no idea what she was doing and appeared to have no control over her actions.

I had become accustomed to Mary's frequent walks, but at three in the morning! Around that time I was awakened by a door slamming shut. After finding that Mary was not in bed I bolted out the door. It was pitch dark when I found Mary roaming about in her nightgown about half a block down the street. Then it started to rain. I had a hard time getting her back to the house. Mary resisted all the way because she wanted to continue her usual walk route.

Mary's *wandering* forced me to install sliding bolts at the top and bottom of the entrance doors for her safety. Fortunately for me, she was unable to reach the top bolt.

INCONTINENCE

One of the most distasteful jobs in caregiving is confronting the *incontinence problem*. It will happen to you eventually, so you might as well be prepared for this necessary task.

Incontinence is divided into two distinct areas: the bladder and the bowels. It is the involuntary release of urine and/or feces.

I remember well my first experience, which was thousands of diaper changes ago. When it first happened I became angry with Mary. It was a stupid reaction on my part. Mary had absolutely no control over her physical functions.

Mary's urinary incontinence started with wetting her pants, the dress she was wearing, and the cushion she was sitting on. When I lifted her to a standing position, a second surge of urine came gushing out all over her legs and shoes, the newly shampooed carpet, as well as my legs and shoes.

In one fell swoop a new crisis was upon me. This was an entirely new and difficult problem to solve—but how?

My last experience with a diaper was with our first child. As a father I was spared most of the diaper changing since Mary did it. Things were different this time: Mary was a hundred-pound woman. In my youth I could evade it. But now I was thrust into it with no real experience. This aspect of my caregiving continued at a rapid pace until her death.

One of my first challenges was to develop a way to prepare Mary for bed that would prevent leaking. I didn't even think about the bed. A kindly nurse advised me to put a diaper on her at bedtime, but as a novice I didn't think to ask her about preparing the bed to protect both Mary and the bed. As usual I had to learn from scratch and fast!

The first night I confidently put the diaper on Mary and tucked her into bed. She went to sleep without any incidents.

But early the next morning when I went to check Mary you wouldn't believe what I found. The stale aroma of urine permeated the room. I hastily threw back the bed covers. *Everything* was soaked with urine: her hair, her body, her nightgown, her diaper, the pillow slip, the pillow cover, the top and bottom bed sheets, the mattress cover, the pillow, and the mattress were reeking with the pungent and penetrating odor of urine. What a mess!

I didn't know whether to laugh or cry. I suppose I did a little of both. In a moment of sheer frustration I opened the bedroom sliding door and threw all of the urine-soaked items, except Mary, onto the lanai and pool deck. They were scattered everywhere. I was sure that no one would ever believe this. I ran into the house, got my camera, and took a picture of this chaotic scene for posterity. Well, posterity is now here. I show this rare picture at the end of the chapter. This one gesture relieved a very stressful moment in my early caregiving.

Mary was such a tiny woman, so where did all the urine come from and what did I do wrong in preparing her for bed? After a lot of investigating I learned a few things.

1. During Mary's thrashing around in the bed her loosely attached diaper separated from her body.

2. There were several actions I should have taken the night before, but didn't.

   • Don't give Mary any liquids after 7 P.M.

   • Buy and use plastic waterproof mattress covers and pillow covers.

   • Buy a waterproof sheet to cover the center of the bed for better protection.

   • Buy large-sized diapers that could be wrapped around her.

   • Use large-sized baby safety pins to secure the legs and stop the leaks.

   • Buy rubber snap-on pants with elastic strips around the legs to put over the diaper.

This was the start of a major change in our life together. It certainly wasn't one I had looked forward to in the "golden years" of retirement.

All of these changes were not accomplished at once. It was a lengthy process of trial and error as necessity warranted. It took a lot of experimenting before I was able to get her incontinent bladder under total control, ending with what I called "dry nights." It was tough but achievable.

But something worse was in store for Mary and me: she became *incontinent of bowel.* For several months Mary was able to sit on the toilet seat, with my help, for her bowel movements. Later she was unable to sit. She would stiffen her back into a prone position and go all over the bathroom floor. Using the toilet for urine and bowel releases was no longer possible.

The obvious answer to this problem was to diaper her twenty-four hours a day. Disposal of the soiled diapers became a problem, but it was quickly solved by using a large plastic trash can with a heavy plastic lining and using liberal amounts of disinfectant spray. The soiled diapers were then picked up twice weekly with the garbage.

The next problem I faced—and it seemed there was always another problem to face—was that of *bowel impaction.* This occurs when the feces becomes hard and cannot be eliminated through normal means of defecation. After all types of laxatives, enemas, oils, and the like were tried but didn't do the job, the ultimate technique called the *digital procedure* had to be used for removal of the impaction. This procedure calls for use of a gloved hand and lubricated finger to enter the anal tract and "dig out" the bowel impaction. To say the least this was a dirty smelly job—but someone had to do it! This procedure does the job well, but it should only be done after consultation and training with a qualified medical specialist.

It was not unusual for me to go through a case and a half of diapers (150–160) monthly. They were used on an as needed basis, usually a minimum of five per day. During Mary's years of dependence on diapers, she used over thirteen thousand. Diapers are costly, so be sure to include them in your medical budget.

One note of caution: long-term use of diapers brings a high risk of *bacterial urinary infection.* The symptoms include a strong urine odor, sweating, elevated temperature, redness of skin in the pubic area, and irritability of patient. It can be treated with antibiotics. The condition is confirmed via laboratory tests and treated with over-the-counter medication. I used a medication called Lotrimin® which did an excellent job for irritation and yeast infections. Close examination of the patient each day will assist in getting the infection under immediate control.

CHOKING

Choking is a characteristic of Parkinson's disease. Mary and I were returning home in our car from an outing. I had some thinly sliced apples in a plastic bag sitting between us in the front seat of the car. I was eating them as we drove and my full attention was focused on the heavy traffic.

In a split second Mary grabbed a slice and put it in her mouth and immediately started to choke. She quickly started turning red and then purple. I swerved the car off the highway onto a narrow strip, raced out my side of the car, opened her door, and reached deep down Mary's throat with my finger and retrieved the slice of apple.

As Mary's color returned to normal and her breathing improved, I was returning to the driver's seat. But before I could sit down Mary had taken another slice of apple and put it in her mouth and once again started to choke. This time I was unable to retrieve the fruit.

Tripler Medical Center was nearby, so I pushed the car to its limit and arrived with Mary at the emergency room, where the good people there retrieved the slice of apple and probably saved her life.

No matter how careful I was when we dined out, the threat of choking always lurked behind the scenes. On one occasion, at a spaghetti restaurant, I had taken great pains to cut Mary's salad into very small pieces. I turned my head for a moment and in that split second Mary grabbed a large piece of lettuce from *my* plate, stuffed it in her mouth, and began to choke. I tried the Heimlich Maneuver but to no avail. She was rapidly turning from red to purple. The manager rushed to call an emergency ambulance. In sheer desperation I thrust my finger deep down her throat and pulled the lodged piece of lettuce out just as the emergency crew arrived. They checked her and found no other problem. This was just one of many such serious incidents which continued and kept me at a constant vigil to the very end of her life.

Choking and aspiration of food (inhaling food) into her lungs became serious threats to Mary's survival. Eventually food had to be processed to a *pureed* texture, using a food processor, then fed to her slowly, a spoonful at a time.

In later stages of her disease phlegm and mucus formed in her throat, which she would try to cough up. This caused new problems. I noticed that the matter would be coughed up into her mouth area then recede back down her throat. To alleviate this problem I obtained a *suction machine,* similar to that used by dentists. This helped to clear her throat and prevent obstructions from entering the lungs. This procedure worked well. Its use should be doctor recommended.

Meal preparation became a precise practice with much care being taken to process Mary's food and develop careful feeding techniques. Choking and the inhaling of food remained constant risks at meal time. Patience was the key while rushing was one of the problems.

Mary's immediate cause of death in 1992 was choking and the aspiration of food into the lungs while in the care of a "care home" during my brief absence.

WANDERING

One day I took Mary with me to the post office. Our son Bob was with us. We all got out of the car and were standing in line to be waited on. Bob returned to the car to pick up another package for mailing. I turned my head away from Mary for a few moments and then turned to speak to her (I thought she was behind me) but she was gone. I immediately started a detailed search around the post office. Bob, who had returned to the post office, ran out to find her, but she had vanished. I continued my search on the street and buildings fronting the post office and beyond. Bob took the route in the back of the building.

After much anguish Bob found Mary nervously pacing back and forth in front of the Kaneohe branch of the Honolulu Savings Bank, one full block away. She had no idea where she was, how she got there, or what she was doing there.

Wandering must be controlled. It's dangerous out there. And it only takes a few seconds to lose sight of your loved one. I would urge you early on to register your patient with a "wanderer's registry" at a local Alzheimer's Association office or with the local police department. Don't forget to get an identification bracelet showing the person's name, disease, and telephone number and secure it on his or her wrist. These preventive measures will assist you in finding your "lost" wanderer.

FORGETTING

Mary had taken her car on an errand. While washing her car that night I noticed a large deep scratch across its entire right side, a scratch that had not been there prior to her trip. When asked she had no idea how or when the scratch got there or where it happened. Curious, I retraced her route and found evidence of her car paint on a guard rail at the entrance to the main highway near our house. She had no idea what I was talking about. After this and other related incidents, her driving career came to an end.

Driving a car is a big responsibility as well as a primary means of independence. The driver must have the capability to react quickly to all driving conditions, since serious or fatal accidents can occur in a flash. When you detect a problem with your relative's driving skills do not hesitate to use all cautionary measures including removing driving privileges for the safety of the patient and others. Removing the driving privileges is a very sensitive action and must be accomplished in a positive rather than a punitive way since you will be taking away another part of the patient's freedom. Handle it lovingly and with a great deal of tact.

The scenes I have described are but a few of the many which occurred during my tenure as a caregiver for Mary. I hope they will give you insight into what you might expect on your watch.

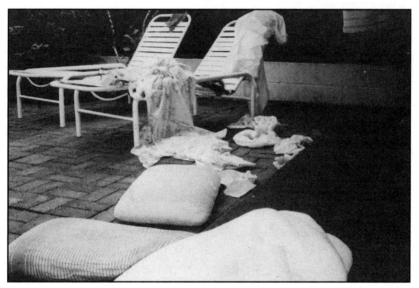

The chaotic "urine scene."

5

Feeding and Nutrition

———⟶•◀———

Feeding was not a problem during the early stages of Mary's disease. However, as her condition progressed problems occurred when she was unable to swallow whole pieces of food, a complication of Parkinson's disease. I first noticed a problem when she was unable to swallow pills. I solved this by giving her the medication with applesauce, which seemed to make the pills go down more easily. This worked well for a long time. Later I needed to grind the pills into granules and combine them with the applesauce. This solved the problem.

Whole foods such as meat, poultry, fish, fruits, and vegetables were prepared the usual way, with the exception of processing them through a *food processor* to obtain a pureed texture that could be fed to Mary slowly with a spoon. Prior to food processing everything on Mary's menu, I would mash all her food with a fork and then cut the meat into very small pieces. This worked, but it was a tedious task. The food processor is the only way to go for this problem.

I would also prepare creative desserts for her. Mary always enjoyed them. I might combine some fruit (bananas, fruit cocktail, peaches, prunes, nuts, etc.) with her favorite chocolate ice cream and process it in the food processor. This was a very healthy concoction which I still use today.

Both Mary and I were on high-fiber and low-cholesterol diets. Lots of fruits and vegetables, skim milk (no eggs or butter), poultry (no fatty meats), and fish. Meats were broiled, not fried.

When I noticed that Mary was beginning to lose weight I consulted the doctor and a nutritionist. I started giving her food supplements. I used a commercial product called Ensure-Plus®, which came in 6 oz. cans. I gave her one can per day up to the time of her death. This product provided her with all the needed nutritional requirements.

Mary also had problems *swallowing* liquids. Swallowing and other functions of the mouth and throat are controlled by a segment of the brain. When that part of the brain is damaged or destroyed, these control functions are weakened or eliminated. When this happens, the liquid flows too fast, restricting normal swallowing. To counter this I used a product called Thick-It®. When added to the liquids such as milk, water, or juice, it would thicken them a bit before I gave them to Mary. This makes it easier for the tongue and throat to process the liquids. This also worked well.

Before resorting to thickeners I was able to give Mary liquids using a straw. Later she was unable to perform the sucking motion to draw the liquid out. This ended the use of straws. At one time I had to use a syringe to squeeze water or juice into Mary's mouth.

The typical meals I would prepare for Mary near the end of her life consisted of:

Breakfast—Orange juice, pureed hot rolled oats with fruit (banana, peaches, fruit cocktail, pears, or other), skimmed milk, unprocessed bran all pureed in the food processor. A glass of Ensure-Plus®. Her medication with applesauce.

Lunch—Apple or cranberry juice. A combination of whole wheat bread, chicken, vegetables with skimmed milk combined into a pureed texture. The content of the food varied from day to day. For dessert I would combine ice cream with fruit (bananas, peaches, pineapple, prunes, or cantaloupe) processed into a pureed texture.

Dinner—Baked potato (then mashed with skim milk), chicken, fish or lean meat (broiled), vegetables (carrots, onions, corn, lima beans, celery, broccoli, cauliflower), or a combination, each pureed. Dinner might also include a salad consisting of lettuce, tomatoes, carrots, cucumbers, onions, celery, and others combined and processed. A glass of Ensure-Plus® food supplement and a dessert similar to one shown for lunch complete dinner.

Snacks—A puree of water, juice, or applesauce combined with graham crackers or cookies.

Medication—Mary had several prescriptions to take daily; most were ground to granules and combined with applesauce. She also took Vitamins A and C daily.

As the disease progressed, her ability to swallow decreased, causing problems receiving food, liquids, and nutrition *into* her body and eliminating waste *from* her body. To enhance normal regularity, be sure to review your patient's food and nutrition intake. Include lots of fruits, juices, natural fiber, and vegetables using a high-fiber diet. Check with a nutritionist for the best diet content for your patient.

Oral Feeding—A speech therapist was recommended for Mary because they are highly skilled in the areas of swallowing, communication, and cognition. They are trained in mouth, oral, and tharyngal (throat) mechanisms, and administer swallowing tests to determine the efficiency of the patient's swallowing mechanisms. Then based on the results of these tests they make appropriate recommendations. After evaluating Mary's condition and ability to ingest food and liquids, a speech therapist from the Rehabilitation Hospital of the Pacific in Honolulu recommended:

1. The safest method would be "non-oral" feeding (use of a nose or stomach tube) because of the high risk of aspiration that is posed by:

   (a) A history of aspiration pneumonia

   (b) Weight loss

   (c) Decreased oral control

   (d) Coughing during meals

   (e) Decreased alertness

2. If oral feeding were to be continued, she recommended that:

   (a) I sit Mary up with her head tilted forward

   (b) All food should be fed by spoon

   (c) I thicken all liquids and reduce solids to puree consistency

   (d) If she coughs, wait at least one minute before continuing

   (e) Monitor her temperature

   (f) I don't feed with a "hot alert"

   (g) I have her sit up for twenty minutes after meals

   (h) I try foods with high calorie content like Ensure-Plus® or Magna Cal® supplements

Near the end of Mary's life the alternatives were essentially two:

1. Insertion of a tube into Mary's stomach as a permanent means of feeding liquids and other vital nutrition into her body.

2. Insertion of a nose tube through the nostril and into the stomach for feeding.

Each method has its advantages and disadvantages. These alternatives were being seriously considered at the time I left Mary at the care home during my short absence in 1992.

I was able to give Mary the meticulous attention needed during her feeding and so I was able to handle it well most of the time. The decision to choose an alternative was not imminent when I left, but one to consider and plan for in the near future.

6

A Pictorial Look at
Mary's Physical Deterioration

—————❖—————

I show on the following pages pictures of Mary taken from 1986 through May 1992. This will allow a better correlation between results and effects of brain degeneration on her body, as discussed in the text, and how it changed Mary's looks over the years of dementia. These pictures graphically identify seven years of dementia's destructive work on Mary's mind and body.

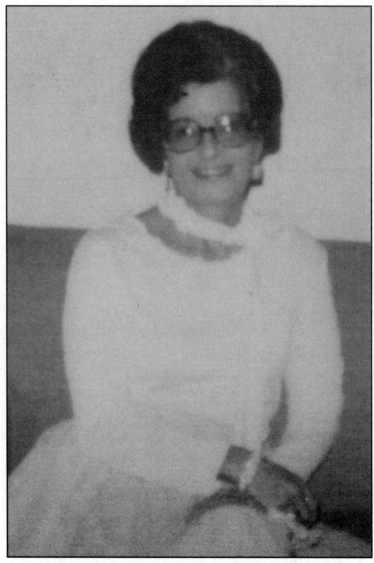

Before the disease and how Mary looked in 1980.

Mary was in excellent health. We had just completed a round of golf. After this photo was taken, we attended a formal military dinner dance at Hickam Air Force Base.

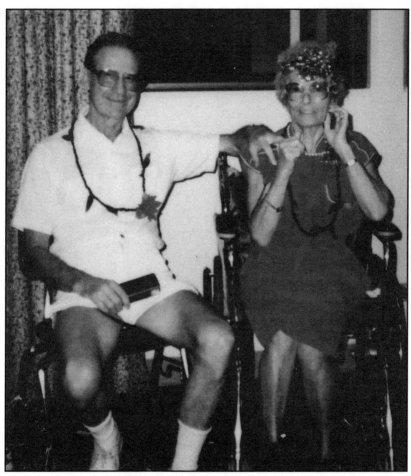

At the Windward Health Center day care in 1986.

I was dropping Mary off at a four-hour experimental respite program given weekly at the center. At this point she was able to speak a little, was incontinent of bladder, and could feed herself with help. You can see her right leg is just starting to contract (involuntarily lift upwards).

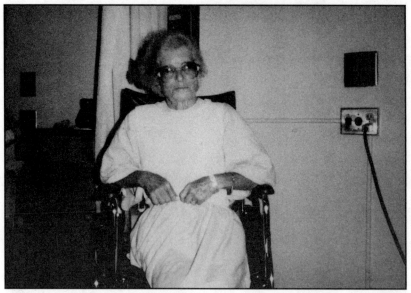

At Tripler Army Medical Center as a patient in 1986.

After several serious falls Mary was admitted to Tripler for treatment and observation. This was her first wheelchair. The only means of securing her in it was a seatbelt, similar to those used in an aircraft. This worked well to transport her from one location to another.

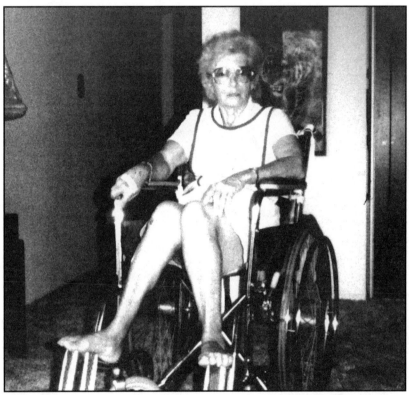

At home in a wheelchair using a "posey restraint" in 1986.

The posey restraint was recommended by the medical staff at Tripler when Mary was discharged. Her use of this restraint is discussed earlier in the book.

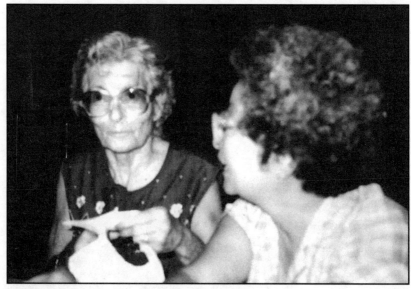

At the Windward Health Center day-care facility in 1987.

Mary is shown with a caregiver as they work on a simple pro-
ject. She was unable to fully comprehend the instructions at this
early stage of her illness.

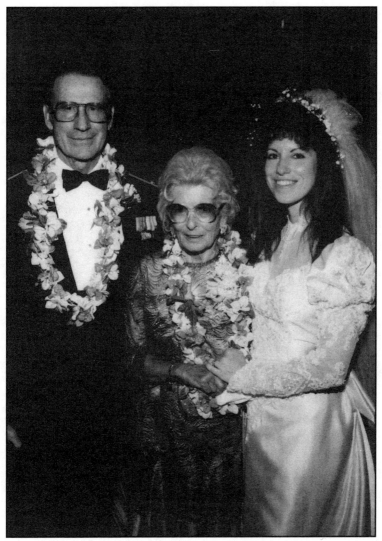

At our daughter Maggie's wedding in 1988.

Mary and I are shown with the bride at her formal wedding in Virginia Beach. We traveled by air from Honolulu to Virginia. Her incontinence and other problems created an extremely challenging trip. This was the last time Mary ever left the island of Oahu!

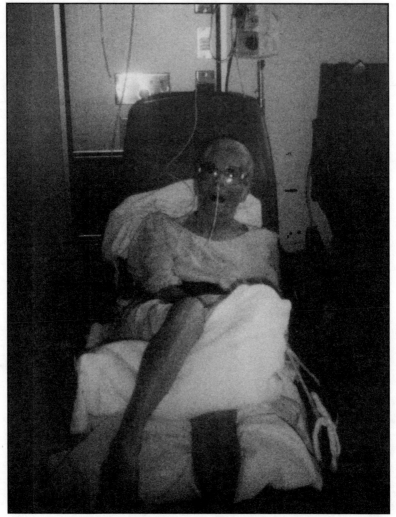

At Tripler Army Medical Center as a patient in 1990.

I was on the mainland for a few days and left Mary at a care facility. During my absence she was admitted to Tripler for dehydration. When notified I immediately returned. The above photo shows Mary with a feeding tube down her nose into her stomach. Her leg was firmly contracted at that time.

The picture below was taken during an outing on the grounds of Tripler Army Medical Center. With a tube in her nose and her mouth open, Mary stares into space. Her hands were beginning to curl and I had inserted rolled wool socks in her hands to counter this action.

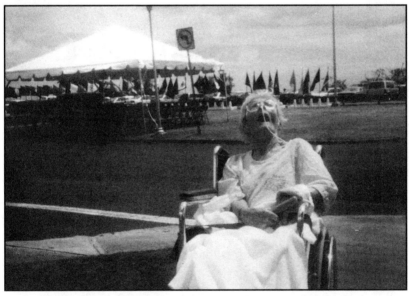

During an outing on the grounds of Tripler Army Medical Center.

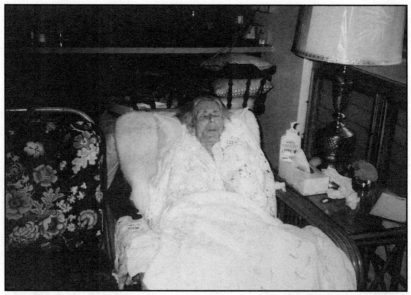

In her seat in the family room on a cold day in 1991.

Mary was made as comfortable as possible in this seat. This is where I fed her pureed food by spoon. I had some of her favorite songs playing softly when she closed her eyes.

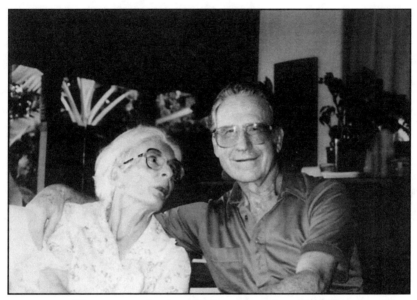

Mary communicating with her eyes on lanai in 1991.

At this stage of her disease Mary was unable to verbally communicate. Her ability to communicate with her hands had also disappeared, but she could communicate with her eyes. It was her last remaining means of letting me know some of her feelings.

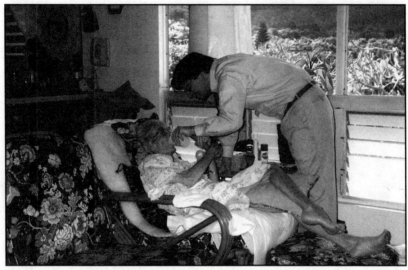

Son Jim (Dr. Wall) tends to Mary in early 1991.

Jim gives Mary a drink of orange juice along with a lot of tender loving care while visiting. Note extended right leg while using pillow between legs to prevent chafing. Also note specially contoured chair making Mary comfortable while preventing her from sliding down.

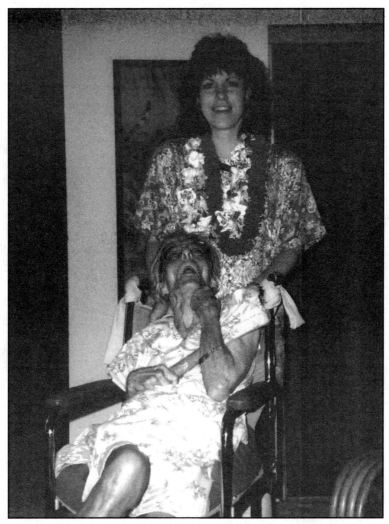

Daughter Maggie visiting from Virginia in mid-1991.

Maggie takes Mary for a wheelchair ride. Although she is unable to talk, Mary is communicating with her eyes, saying, "Let's get the show on the road." Note her right hand clutching a handgrip, her open mouth, contracted right leg, and an Alzheimer's identification bracelet on her left arm.

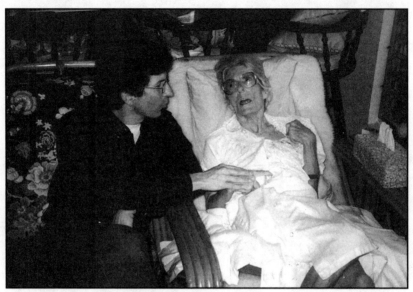

Son Bob visiting from Brazil in late 1991.

Bob talks to Mary while holding her hand. Mary is unable to communicate verbally but responds with a quizzical look and communicates with her eyes. Note open mouth, handgrips, and curled left wrist.

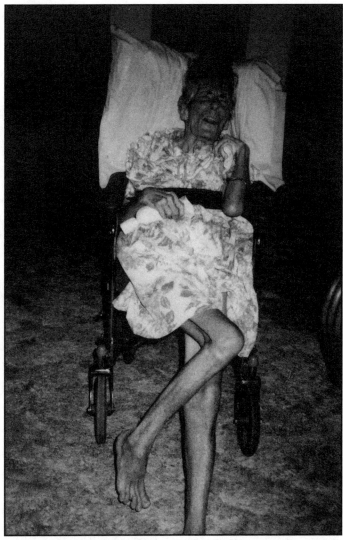

In her wheelchair at home in mid-1992.

Note Mary's inability to sit up straight, the worsening of her contracted right leg, and use of handgrips in each hand to prevent curling and digging into her flesh. This was in the last stage of her disease.

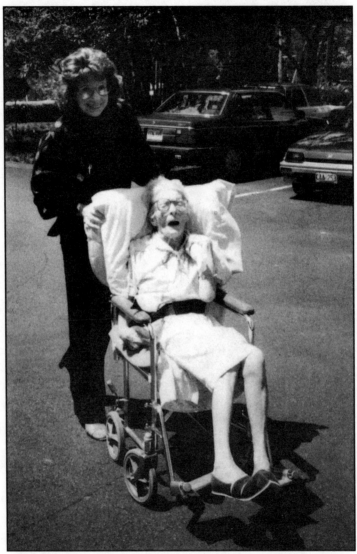

Out for an outing in her small-wheeled wheelchair in 1992.

My sister Jeanette is taking Mary for a ride in Haiku Gardens near our home. She loved these rides and the beautiful mountainous terrain. This is how she looked a few months before her death.

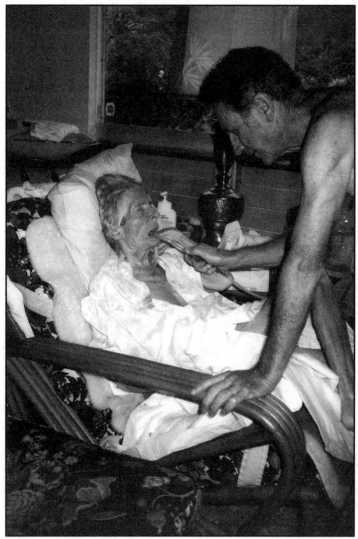

Having matter extracted from her throat using a suction machine in mid-1992.

Mary in her seat in the family room when she needed her throat cleared to prevent choking. I used this suction machine to suck out the matter and clear her throat. This was a very effective medical aid. I started using this a few months before her death.

Mary loved her seat on the lanai overlooking the fantastically beautiful mountain setting which was the background behind the swimming pool she also loved. I wanted to have her in "her chair" one more time. It was Mary's wish to be cremated upon her death. The cremation was accomplished on July 23, 1992. Her remains were placed in the urn selected by our family. We stopped to bring Mary "home" and to take her picture at the place she loved for the last time.

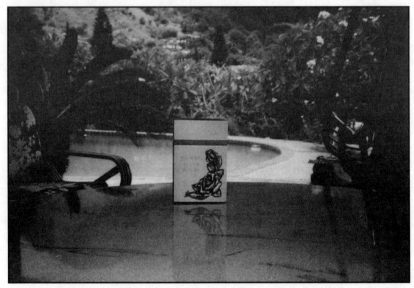

In her final resting place in her urn en route to the inurnment site on July 24, 1992.

7

The Hard Facts of Life

"Mary has an *incurable disease* that will result in her death." I was sitting in front of the doctor in his office when I was confronted with this terrifying statement. How was I to handle this problem? I tried to ask all the right questions only to learn that there are no right answers. My inner voice rebelled, saying, "I don't believe it. Don't worry, you always got out of difficult situations before and you can do it now. We'll find a way."

Then later the doctor handed me a second blast: "The only thing we can do for Mary is to make her as comfortable as possible; further medication is ineffective." The shock was indescribable. Inside I was devastated. I soon learned that "progressive" meant Mary's illness would be on a one-way destructive path at various speeds—depending on many factors—with no turning back. I also learned that "irreparable" meant that the part of Mary's brain that was destroyed could not be repaired and would never again be able to direct the functions of mind and body formerly controlled by the destroyed brain cells.

At an early stage of Mary's disease the use of the medication Sinemet® worked wonders for the Parkinson's side of her illness. However, with the passing of time this healing drug became less useful and finally useless. This was another hard fact to confront.

If I became sick, I still had to care for Mary. She had to come first. She depended on me for everything every day. As the saying goes, "I didn't have the time to be sick."

During my caregiving for Mary I was seldom sick. Tired and worn out, yes. I was always able to tend to her needs. When I had a doctor's appointment I would try to arrange to have someone to sit with Mary or I would take her to a day care or a respite center for a few hours. Sometimes I just took her with me when she was able to do so. I had one real emergency situation when I became extremely dizzy at 3 A.M. I was unable to stand or walk. My foremost thought was "What about Mary?" From my bed I tried to stand up but my head was spinning. I managed to place my hands against the wall and shuffle along the walls to the bathroom and to the telephone. I called another caregiver friend who came to tend Mary. I then called a neighbor who took me to the emergency room at Tripler Army Medical Center. This was a harrowing experience that really scared me.

Arrangements always had to be made for the patient first under all circumstances. I was caring for a fragile human life. My problems had to be secondary to Mary's needs.

There were so many hard facts to face about the quality of Mary's life during those last years. With each new limitation it seemed as though I had reached my limit. I couldn't bear any more. But then I'd think of a way to overcome the problem and we would move on. It seemed I was being controlled by the proverbial carrot on the stick: I tried my best but it was never quite enough. When I would face a new obstacle, I'd find myself saying: "Not this. How can they do this to Mary? I'll show them." The biggest setbacks in my quest to help Mary proved to be her inability to talk, walk, use the toilet (incontinence), shower, dress, groom, and feed herself, and to perform dental and body hygiene and the other normal functions of living.

As one ability after another was taken away from her, I found myself experiencing an emotional reaction to each. Had I not been able to control my anger and frustration at this devastating disease, the consequences for my own health and well-being could have been considerable.

In addition to watching the daily deterioration of Mary's malfunctioning mind and body, I deeply resented that *our* time together—our retirement—was being ruthlessly taken away. We would never again:

- Dance together—one of our passions
- Go on long walks in the hills and mountains or wade and swim at the beautiful beaches
- Experience the passion and joy of sexual intimacy
- Enjoy traveling all over the country and the world
- Go to restaurants, shows, the theater, play golf, and attend athletic events
- Enjoy meeting old and new friends for a night out
- Live as healthy people do and enjoy life to the fullest
- Have the love and companionship we enjoyed in the past

These are some of the ways Multi-infarct-dementia, Parkinson's, and Alzheimer's steal our loved ones from us, leaving little more than a shell of a person. Caregiving is a tough assignment.

But the hardest thing to face in this whole saga had to be the frantic telephone call I received in Virginia from the head nurse at the care home in Kailua, Hawaii, on July 19, 1992, giving me the shocking news that "Mary is dead"!

8

Mary Confronts Her Disease

Mary's reactions to her illness ranged from disbelief to a determination to deal with it. At other times she simply wasn't able to understand or comprehend the enormity of its fury, the rapidity of its growth, or the consequences of its destructive power. Here I will try to describe some of her reactions to the various milestone incidents as they occurred during the different stages of her disease.

When symptoms started to become more pronounced, Mary's first reaction was to tell me, "I know there is something wrong with me, but I'm sure I can handle it, so don't worry." But as the disease progressed, there would be times when Mary would look up at me and say in a slow, pleading voice, "What is happening to me? I'm losing my mind."

On the golf course putting green when she *fell* for the first time, I recall her saying, "It's nothing, let's continue to play." Here she showed the courage and gutsy attitude that would sustain her during the time she was still able to react mentally and verbally to the increasingly severe limitations on her mind and body.

One Sunday morning while seated at the kitchen bar eating breakfast, Mary turned to me and said, "I'm going to *faint.*" I carried her to the couch and laid her down. After a few minutes she got up and was back to normal. This same scenario was repeated at exactly the same time and location one week later, resulting in the same words and actions. We found out later these episodes were the start of her ministrokes.

Once during a football game at Aloha Stadium in Honolulu, Mary excused herself to go to the ladies room. I felt confident she could go and return with no problems. I was wrong. On this occasion the stadium was packed with over fifty thousand people milling about. After fifteen minutes Mary had not returned. I went to the ladies rest room and asked a woman entering if she would check to see if Mary was in there. She checked and advised me Mary was not there. I began to panic. How was I to find a small grey-haired lady in a capacity crowd?

I went back into the area overlooking the stadium and was scanning the entire arena, when I noticed a lady of Mary's description about three sections away (a quarter of the length of the stadium). I raced down to find Mary searching for our seats. I had done the impossible—I found the needle in the haystack! She had made a wrong turn, became disoriented, and got lost.

You'll recall that I mentioned that Mary had taken a serious fall on our tiled bathroom floor. She hit her head so hard that we had to visit the hospital emergency room for stitches to close the wound on her forehead. When the doctor administered a shot into the wound to kill the pain, Mary reacted with a loud clear "OUCH!" That was the last time I ever heard her speak a word.

Mary would often react to soft classical music. She would respond to it with her eyes. I would play tapes or records of her old favorite songs: "Let Me Call You Sweetheart," "Ave Maria," "Be My Love," "White Christmas," and "I'll Be Seeing You." She seemed to look forward to the relaxing softness of the music.

At one stage of her illness Mary had an obsession for trying to get up. She would not stay seated. She seemed to have an over-powering urge to get up immediately once seated, as if something she didn't like was going to happen and she wanted to stop it. Later she reacted in the same manner toward falling. Whenever she fell she would immediately try to stand only to fall again.

I would take her on daily wheelchair rides, weather permitting. At the beginning she would sit upright and genuinely enjoy the beautiful scenery near the majestic Koolau Mountains in Kaneohe, Hawaii. She savored the view and the soft tropical breeze on her face and body. But as the disease progressed, her ability to sit up straight in the wheelchair degenerated to the point where she would half sit-half lie in the wheelchair in a stiff horizontal position with a glazedlike stare into space as if in another world.

It was extremely difficult to determine the extent to which Mary was able to understand what was going on in her mind and body and specifically how she felt about her illness. Sometimes I was sure I could read signals she seemed to be sending from her eyes. Mary's *eyes* had become an important means of communication between us.

When I went out to the pool her eyes would try to follow me. When I was on the pool deck looking at her through the window her eyes were telling me, "Don't worry, everything is okay." When I entered a room after an absence she would tell me with her eyes how glad she was to see me. When I fed her pureed food by the spoonful her eyes would say, "Thank you, I needed that." And on those all too frequent occasions when she had a bowel impaction requiring a digital procedure to remove the obstruction, her eyes would change from pain and anticipation to total relief after the procedure. Soon thereafter another eye communication would be saying to me, "Boy, that sure did make me feel better. Thanks."

When I could, I would take Mary to the Hale Koa Hotel in Waikiki for dinner, since it was easy to park and enter. I would always get a booth, take her from the wheelchair and prop her in a corner of the booth, and then park the wheelchair, hoping all the while that she would not fall. This procedure usually worked great but there were exceptions.

On one occasion I was sporting a cast on my left forearm. I had fractured the arm while tending Mary. I seated her as usual and went to park the wheelchair. When I returned I found Mary lying in a prone position on the floor under the table. "Mary, what are you doing under there?" I asked. With her silent speech, Mary's sheepish half-grin looked back at me as if to say, "I don't know how I got down here, but just get me up."

I can't deny that these short trips required considerable effort to plan and carry out, but they were worth it just to get both of us out of the house for a short time. The added bonus was that I didn't have to prepare dinner that night. These little trips could be a brief respite for both of us.

After she could no longer speak, Mary would react with hand signals. I would ask her a question and request her to respond by squeezing my hand. This worked well for a while. Later her hands were tightly closed and eventually curled into a fist, negating even this means of communication.

During the last months of her life Mary's body reacted to her multiple diseases in a retrograde manner. Her right leg was contracted, elevated, and stiff; her hands were curled; and at times it seemed as if she were returning to the fetus position of birth.

During the last year of her life Mary was unable to react to anything or control any of her mental or physical functions. If the Mary I knew and loved was still with me, she was buried deep within the stiffened joints and muscles of a body that could no longer react to stimulation, and her mind was confined to a brain that continually underwent the degenerating attacks of stroke, Parkinson's, and Alzheimer's. Her silence spoke volumes.

9

How the Disease
Affected the Family

Mary's disease had a very profound effect on our whole family. Most immediately its impact was felt by Mary and me. We both felt cheated that what were to be the best years of our lives had been devastated by a set of circumstances over which we had no control. The days of leisure and contentment were stolen from us.

Our three children were scattered throughout the world. The eldest son, Bob, works and lives in Brazil, while another son, Jim, is a doctor with a practice in Oklahoma. Our daughter, Maggie, works and lives in Virginia with her family. Mary's twin sister, Margaret, lives in California, while Mary and I were living in Hawaii. We are a very close-knit family, but through the years the normal relationships of family closeness have not been possible due to the tremendous distances that separate us. Family members were unable to perform any personal care for Mary, except on infrequent visits. However, they were very supportive in providing moral assistance through frequent letters and telephone calls. My son the doctor provided medical advice on care for which I was very grateful.

Mary's total dependence on my caregiving caused a complete change in our lifestyle. Everything was now focused on one primary concern, the health and welfare of my wife. It was a round-the-clock responsibility with no holidays.

During the early days of the illness our lifestyle didn't change significantly. We could still talk (with some patience), go places, and do things with friends. Socializing became less frequent as friends who were close in the past seemed to shy away due to their uneasiness when trying to converse with Mary or their inability to cope with her disease.

I met several new friends while attending classes, briefings, seminars, and meetings given by the Alzheimer's Association, support groups, hospitals, and local government-sponsored programs. I met Carl Tapfer, who is mentioned in the Acknowledgments, in the basement of a parking lot at an Alzheimer's respite center in Honolulu as we both struggled with our loved ones to get them out of the car and into their wheelchairs and then into the center so we could have a three- or four-hour reprieve from our demanding caregiver tasks.

This new set of friends, many of whom were struggling with similar problems, shared values and concerns. It was great just talking on the phone. They were not concerned with Mary's appearance or condition. They were genuine friends and had a therapeutic effect on me. Whether they realized it or not, these special people helped a lot. As Mary's disease progressed and its toll on both of us was mounting, my new goal was to treat Mary with love and patience while keeping her clean and comfortable. Sometimes all seemed to be lost, but I had to try.

A retired air force colonel, the military had trained me to do many things, but none touched on the techniques of caregiving. This was a tough way to learn—on the job and under pressure.

As Mary's primary caregiver my life was affected in many ways both mental and physical. During every minute of the day, Mary had to be uppermost in my thoughts and actions. My social life was essentially forfeited. Our sex life was nonexistent. Of necessity, in the course of normal and emergency conditions, I found myself performing the functions of doctor, nurse, occupational therapist, feeder, diaper changer, bather, house cleaner, family coordinator, banker, and investor, in addition to one-sided conversationalist, pool care technician, gardener, landscaper, and many others.

Mary's frequent falls and bouts with choking forced me to become an expert in lifesaving. I also became accomplished at administering medication to a person who doesn't want to take it. I had to prepare and brief the doctors on the status of Mary's condition in a concise and factual manner, which was then used as the basis for treatment. Having been trained in briefing techniques, I could handle it, but this meant I had to learn the new medical vocabulary related to these diseases.

I didn't have time to be sick; however, time and events sometimes took their toll on my well-being. At first I thought I could do the whole job by myself, but as I gradually reached the tolerance threshold—my emotional and physical breaking point—I realized how wrong I was.

I learned early on that I was going to need help in caring for Mary. I initially went to Alzheimer's Association support group meetings, where I met other caregivers and guest speakers who passed on their experiences and recommended other activities and people to contact. I also attended several briefings, meetings, and seminars on the various diseases of dementia conducted by city and state health departments and hospitals. I learned a lot about caregiving from these, but the real teacher was the actual experience of caregiving. I would take any respite I could get. Sometimes I would get respite and relief when due to Mary's rapid deterioration she needed a higher level of care. Sometimes I felt spent and actually became sick. However, I was totally responsible for Mary's daily well-being and this took precedence. Looking at her I decided she was suffering more than I, so my sickness became secondary.

I notice the emotional drain continues as I recall these past incidents while preparing this book, but doing this also has its therapeutic rewards as it transfers deep-rooted feelings from within to a written chronology of happenings.

Our children felt a great personal loss when their mother became ill. She had been their provider and their emotional anchor while I was on unaccompanied military assignments. Mary provided them with love, comfort, and guidance. She raised each of them to be strong, disciplined, healthy, and successful citizens. They expressed their love for their mother in many ways by their actions during visits: feeding her, talking to her, holding her hands, taking her for wheelchair rides. They also sent her flowers and other presents and encouraging letters and cards for me to read to her. Her illness and death tragically brought home the fact that neither she nor I would always be there for them.

Mary's sister, Margaret, had mixed reactions to Mary's illness. As children they were inseparable, and with age they remained very close, confiding in each other. They depended on each other with an emotional intimacy that only twins share. Margaret's emotional pain was evident, as was her quest for details about Mary's illness. Understandably, Margaret feared that this tragic illness could also target her. She experienced the great loss of a loved one with whom she realized a closeness beyond sibling bonding. An important part of her life no longer exists, and it has left a large void that will never be filled.

Mary's illness brought her family members closer to each other as they reaffirmed the importance of family love and togetherness.

10

The Humor Approach Helps

Caregiving is an extremely serious undertaking, one in which life-and-death decisions sometimes have to be made. However, there are times when the most serious situations have a very humorous dimension. If you look at it from this point of view, you will find it relieves stress while you enjoy the funny side of an otherwise stressful event.

I would like to share with you now some of the funnier incidents that occurred while tending to Mary's needs.

In 1988, Mary and I were en route to our daughter Maggie's wedding. The aircraft was making its final approach heading for Norfolk, Virginia, when Mary's diaper was in need of being changed. New mothers no doubt have quite a time seeing to the needs of a baby on board a commercial aircraft, so you can imagine my challenge trying to change a one-hundred-pound woman's diaper in a small lavatory at the tail end of the plane while coming in for a landing in a high crosswind, the tail wagging and Mary squirming. I had only two hands, but I needed three. I was smiling as I struggled to help Mary back to our seats. One flight attendant watching me said, "Bless you." The trip with Mary was a calculated risk, but it was worth it. She was able to witness her only daughter get married.

On another occasion I was taking Mary for a walk, during an early stage of her illness at which she could not stand up alone. She could still move her left leg, however. I would get behind her, placing my right foot under her right foot, and we would hobble along. It helped me to exercise her legs. I'm sure we looked quite a sight shuffling down the street. People would stop their cars to encourage me. Some would give the "thumbs up" sign while others would toot their car horns and throw in a "Bless you" or other encouraging remarks. They made me feel much better in an invigorating sort of way.

Some of the many humorous incidents that occurred while caring for Mary were highlighted in my 1989 Christmas letter sent to our family and friends throughout the country. Their positive response to these annual letters on Mary was another factor in my decision to write this book.

"ALOHA" and "MELE KALIKIMAKA"—1989

(From the Walls)

This year for the Walls was one of "education and patience."

It happened in 1989. We did not make a trip to anywhere, except to the bathroom, hospitals, clinics, doctor's offices, emergency rooms, day-care centers, pharmacies, and the like.

The year was completed without the execution of our projected plans to visit friends and relatives in San Francisco and Virginia Beach, Virginia, which were cancelled due to Mary's deteriorating condition.

Education is continuous in life, from birth to death. You learn something every day. For example, my eight years of college and all my years in the military and in business did not prepare me for what has been the learning experience of my life during the past three years.

Of necessity I've become a nurse, pharmacist, doctor, diaper changer, feeder, bather, hair dresser, shopper, house cleaner, cook, food buyer, dresser, groomer, companion, clothes selector, decision maker, banker, investor, contortionist, and one-sided conversationalist.

Humor is a must if I am to survive in this buzz-saw business of caregiving. Several incidents occurred which I'd like to share with you:

At San Francisco Airport Mary's diaper needed changing, so into the men's room we went with one diaper and two safety pins. We found a stall and I started to change Mary. While I was work-ing with one pin, I put the other needed safety pin on the toilet paper dispenser. At a critical time, with Mary's arms flailing, the safety pin was brushed into the next stall under a guy's foot! As I slowly reached under the stall to retrieve the pin, all the while try-ing to balance Mary with my other hand, someone stepped on my hand! Ah, well, who needs the damn pin. Let the diaper fall, right?

In Kaneohe, Hawaii, I took Mary for a walk (actually, more like a drag). While entering an area with other people and a dog, Mary couldn't move. When I looked down I saw that her diaper had fallen to her ankles and watched two small BMs roll out. Quickly I pulled up her diaper, looked at the people, and blamed it (the BMs) on the dog.

During another walk with Mary in Kaneohe I had forgotten to zip up the front of my walking shorts. At one point Mary tripped, her elbow unbuttoned the top button of my shorts, and, you guessed it, my shorts fell down in the middle of the busy street. Passing motorists looked, others laughed, and some even stopped to aid me. Hell, I didn't need help, just patience!

In the bathroom shower with my fractured left wrist bone in a cast with a plastic cover over it, I had Mary propped in the shower (she stands on her left toes with her right leg in the air). Just as she was all clean and ready to get out, she drops two big BMs and simultaneously puts her right foot down hard closing the drain, while a spray of soapsuds is squirted into both of my eyes.

A caregiver must be a good planner. Everything must be in place before I make a move to the bathroom: diapers, wipes, safety pins, tape, baby oil, powder, golashes, underthings, outer garments . . .

Mary has a pretty smile. She recognizes me. She depends on me for everything. We sing old songs each day while driving to the day-care center. Our theme song is "Let Me Call You Sweetheart." She can't talk or generate voice conversation—but she can hum along with the "Oldies" sometimes. Strange this thing called dementia.

Our Christmas Message for 1989: Time is of the essence, do what you're planning today. Keep healthy, eat well, exercise regularly, and be kind to each other. Life is short but precious even with its adversities. We send our love to each of you. Till we meet again in 1990! Your friends—

Mary   Andy/Frank

11

Who Takes Care of the Caregiver?

⟢⟡⟣

The answer to this question is simple. Caregivers must take care of themselves! A caregiver is anyone who sees to the needs of another. The duties vary in type, scope, and complexity. The person needing care could be a spouse, an elderly parent, or any other family member.

Usually caregivers are pressed into service by necessity under crisis or adverse financial conditions, rarely by choice. Sometimes the tasks sound easy at first but caregiving is a highly complex adventure that takes a heavy toll on the mental and physical well-being of the provider.

Not only is caregiving complex, frustrating, and costly, but it can quickly turn into a total dependence relationship of the patient on the caregiver, as was my relationship with Mary. This total dependence of one human being on another for basic daily needs is an awesome burden for anyone to carry.

In order to perform this formidable task, caregivers must maintain their mental and physical health at optimal levels. I quickly learned the type, scope, and variety of demands Mary's illness would place on me. I had to take immediate inventory of my own assets and state of health, my existing commitments, my eating and exercise habits, and devise a plan to handle the job as best I could. It's always wise to get a complete physical examination to determine from a medical standpoint physical strengths and deficiencies. Then in coordination with a doctor or counselor, develop realistic diet and exercise programs tailored to meet your specific needs. Religiously follow the program.

If your cholesterol is high (above 200), you need to modify your diet. There are two types of cholesterol: LDL is the bad one which deposits a waxy buildup called plaque on the walls of your arteries. This impairs blood flow and can lead to heart attack or stroke. HDL is the good one which carries cholesterol out of the bloodstream.

LDL can be controlled by diet. Cutting down on saturated fats (animal products including milk, eggs, cheeses, organ and fatty cuts of meats, and the like) will help to lower this cholesterol.

HDL can be increased by a good exercise program. (Its normal range is 35+). Exercise also increases your cardiovascular fitness since the heart is a muscle that becomes bigger and stronger through exercise and its increasing demand for oxygen. This kind of exercise is called "aerobics." You should also consider walking, swimming, jogging, or calisthenics as good candidates for an exercise program.

The American Heart Association located in your community has all the details on both the HDL and LDL programs. Contact them and get into a wellness program now. You are going to need it in your stressful role as caregiver. Such a program helped me survive my seven-year ordeal with Mary's illness. Remember, *your* health is vital to the survival of your patient.

To survive in the fast-track environment of caregiving you must also look to the element of humor to maintain your objectivity. Look on the light side of everything you do, especially when interacting with your patient. Smilers are winners, whiners are losers. Be a winner. Always display love and compassion with kind words and actions; it will cause surprising things to happen to you and to your patient.

Keep in contact with your family members for assistance or help in any way they can give it: financial, physical, or just plain moral support. Never turn down any offers to help. Depending on them is what the family is all about. "Pride," "revenge," "guilt," and "recrimination" are words that should be stricken from your vocabulary and your mind. You don't have time to indulge in such matters.

Use any free time to the maximum—for you! Get out with friends, play golf, go to the beach, go hiking, exercise, or just relax. But remember to focus your attention on what free time means—a respite for you. You'll return to caregiving refreshed and renewed.

I looked in the phone book for "Alzheimer's Association." They gave me a list of support groups in my area. I also attended one of their meetings and was able to bring Mary in a wheelchair. They cared for her during the meeting. This provided me with a short respite period as a bonus. They also had information about other meetings that would help. Alzheimer's chapters are everywhere throughout the United States.

Seek out and attend support group meetings. Participate by getting your frustrations out into an open forum of your peers, many of whom probably have experienced more devastating problems and have found some encouraging solutions to some of your problems. This vital therapy is there for the taking.

Keep a diary of events as they occur when caring for your loved one. Be sure to make the entries time-sensitive, accurate, and legible. This data can be used later as a basis for developing articles or other public information materials or just to have a personal chronicle of significant events in the progression of the disease as well as the thoughts and feelings of both you and your loved one. At some point this record could be given to family members as a historical/medical record. This also provides you with an outlet for your stress and emotions while providing something valuable for your family. This writing process helped me capture my thoughts and release some of my deep feelings during periods of intense stress.

Try to avoid isolation. As a caregiver your lifestyle has drastically changed and your energy reserves (such as they are) are not usually up to the demands of socializing. Now that you are no longer a "twosome" your old friends seem to fade away, which can leave you feeling discouraged and sorry for yourself. This is a good time to seek new friends who have common interests with you and the person to whom you are giving care. Support group meetings are an excellent place to develop new friendships or just provide someone to talk to on the phone about your caregiver problems. Don't overlook renewing ties with your church. The congregation will provide much-needed spiritual and human support through fellowship, friendship, and church-sponsored programs and resources.

Don't become a *casualty* of your patient's disease. It's easy to do, especially if you disregard the warning signs. When you feel you are getting out of control, seek counseling. The first step is *always* the hardest, but think of the alternatives!

Don't become a victim of *stress*. As a caregiver you are a high-risk candidate. You should be aware of the warning signs of burn-out and stress, which include:

- Intestinal distress
- Frequent illness
- Anxiety
- Outbursts of anger
- Feeling overwhelmed
- Increased irritability (conflicts with family or others)
- Rapid pulse
- Insomnia
- Depression
- Persistent fatigue
- Lack of concentration
- Increased use of alcohol, drugs, or caffeine

You shouldn't ignore these signs of stress. Discuss them with your family, your doctor, or a counselor. With their help you may learn some of the ways to cope with stress, such as the following:

- Try not to worry about things you cannot control.

- Practice relaxation techniques like deep breathing and deliberately relaxing specific sets of muscles in an orderly progression.

- Limit your intake of alcohol, drugs, and caffeine.

- Make time for recreation and respite.

- Exercise regularly. Walking is a good start.

- Redefine your professional and personal expectations so they are realistic and achievable.

- Learn to say *no*: set limits and maintain personal boundaries.

- Resolve conflicts in ways that don't force you to suppress your feelings.

- When in conflict with someone, try to find solutions that meet your needs as well as those of the person with whom you are in conflict.

When stress is out of control it prevents caregivers from effectively performing their duties. Take time to understand and react when the signs of stress are evident in your life. Caregivers and stress seem to go together naturally, but don't let stress get beyond your ability to control it.

I found that researching in the library, studying, and attending seminars and lectures about Mary's illness, rather than totally depending on infrequent doctor's visits, gave me a better mental attitude and a clearer understanding of the diseases and better prepared me to more intelligently discuss her symptoms and reactions and progress or deterioration with the physician. This also helped the doctor in his evaluations and treatments in addition to reducing my levels of stress and emotion during the visits. As a twenty-four-hour caregiver, you will know more about the patient than the doctor. However, you must be prepared to update the doctor on status and changes as they occur.

Remember, you are the only one who can really take care of the caregiver. By making your own physical and emotional needs a priority you will be in a better position to serve the one who needs your care.

12

How the End Came

On July 19, 1992, while I was in Virginia visiting our daughter and on a long delayed and much-needed respite vacation, I received a frantic telephone call from the care home in Kailua, Hawaii, where Mary was being cared for during my brief absence. The head nurse, in an emotionally charged voice, chokingly blurted out, "Mary didn't make it! She just didn't make it!" I anxiously responded, "What do you mean? What happened?" The nurse then said, *"Mary is dead!"* Even though I had watched Mary's illness take her from me bit by bit and for some time I had lost the woman I knew as wife and mother, friend and lover, the news still came as a huge shock.

The cause of death was listed as *accidental.* The immediate cause of death was "aspiration of food" and the contributing cause was "Parkinson's disease." All of this was reflected in the official autopsy report conducted by the medical examiner of the City and County of Honolulu and recorded on the official death certificate issued by the state of Hawaii. An accidental death in the state of Hawaii requires that a mandatory autopsy be performed on the deceased.

A chronology of the feverish preparations made for Mary's temporary care home stay and the details of her death were noted in my 1992 Christmas letter to friends and relatives. It was entirely devoted to Mary.

"ALOHA" and "MELE KALIKIMAKA"—1992

(From the Walls)

This year was not a good one for the Walls. It is with a heavy heart that I must write the final tribute to Mary and discuss how the end came—but first I will restate for you the "Last Prayer for Mary" prepared and given by me at her "Inurnment" at Punch Bowl National Cemetery in Honolulu, Hawaii, on July 24, 1992.

THE LAST PRAYER FOR MARY WALL

The Lord reached out his arms for Mary and she left for the unknown on July 19, 1992.

Mary was a loving, caring wife and a dedicated and devoted mother. As a long-time volunteer she continually helped those less fortunate.

I grieve her loss as a companion and friend of forty-nine years, but rejoice that she is relieved of her years of suffering against overwhelming odds and is now in the hands of a higher power.

God Bless you Mary. I love you.

Your Husband, Andy

HOW THE END CAME

Mary's serious condition continued to deteriorate rapidly during 1992. It became extremely difficult to cope with the old and all the new problems that continually occurred, all of which weakened her ability to react and survive.

As Mary's primary caregiver I was very close to "burn out" in late June 1992. I just had to take a break and get off the island. Then came the nagging questions: What about Mary? Will she be okay? Where do I take her? Will they care for her like I do?

After painstaking and meticulous research and preparation I selected a care home to take care of Mary during my absence. Then the preparation work really began: doctor's appointments for Mary, updating the doctor on Mary's status, preparing written instructions for Mary's required care, getting the needed medications, procuring all the supplies for two weeks (diapers, etc.), packing her things, getting Mary ready, and then delivering her to the care home. What a job.

Second thoughts on leaving Mary continually flashed across my mind. Should I leave her? What if . . . ? Can she survive without me? I had confidence in the care home which I had used on a similar trip in 1991. The hard decision was made; now I just had to go.

So away I went, very tired but with feelings of relief, some anxiety, and, yes, guilt. First I flew to California for a visit with Mary's twin sister, Margaret, and her husband. Then I flew on to Baltimore for a visit with son Jim, followed by a trip to Virginia Beach for a visit with daughter Maggie and family. During each stop I would call the care home, whose staff would always report "Mary is doing fine." However, on July 19, after being out late that evening I received a frantic telephone call from the head nurse at the care home. She blurted out, "Mary didn't make it! She just didn't make it!" I anxiously responded, "What do you mean? What happened?" She said, "Mary is dead!"

Mary was being fed breakfast, and the last spoonful of pureed cereal in the bowl had just been given to her. She started to swallow, but the food was going down the wrong way (into the lungs). She could not generate enough strength to cough up the food. The food had aspired into her lungs, cutting off the oxygen to her brain and resulting in heart failure. It was a quick end. Mary left us at that moment. The death certificate shows the cause of her death as accidental!

Maggie returned with me to Hawaii on the next available flight out of Virginia. Jim flew in from San Diego, where he was on vacation, and surprisingly met us at Honolulu Airport. Bob flew in from Brazil the next day. Once again the Wall family of five were together again, for the last time.

Funeral arrangements were made in record time. After a brief ceremony for family and friends, Mary was inurned at the National Memorial Cemetery of the Pacific (Punch Bowl) in Honolulu, Hawaii.

And now for the Christmas message for 1992. We are on this earth only on a temporary basis: we are born, we grow and prosper, and we die. Time is not only of the essence, it is a precious commodity and should not be thrown away or wasted. Forget bitterness, procrastination, revenge, discrimination, etc. Be thankful for your time on earth. Use it wisely.

Remember now, do it today, tomorrow may be too late. Give your spouse a great big hug and kiss and say, "Honey, I love you." Be good to each other because it's tough to be alone! Till we meet again in 1993.

ANDY/FRANK

13

The Last Prayer for Mary

━━━➤⊷⊶◄━━━

I composed this last prayer and delivered it at Mary's Inurnment
at the National Memorial Cemetery of the Pacific (Punch Bowl)
in Honolulu, Hawaii, on July 24, 1992.

"The Last Prayer for MARY McARTHUR WALL"

(Free at Last)

**The Lord reached out his arms for MARY
and she left for the unknown on July 19, 1992.**

Mary was a loving, caring wife and
a dedicated and devoted mother.
As a long-time volunteer she continually
helped those less fortunate.

I grieve her loss as a companion
and friend of forty-nine years,
but rejoice that she is relieved of
her years of suffering against
overwhelming odds and is now
in the hands of a higher power.

God Bless you Mary—I love you.

Your Husband, Andy

14

Lessons Learned

——⊷◈⊷——

I endured a very stressful period during my seven years as a caregiver for Mary. It was a combination of emotions:

- *Happiness*—being able to help my loved one through the traumatic and difficult times.

- *Frustration*—in not understanding the real implications and scope of her illness.

- *Elation*—when a new procedure or medication relieved some of her pain and suffering.

- *Disappointment*—when nothing was helping or stopping critical mental and physical changes rapidly taking place in Mary, while I could only stand back and watch the deterioration happen.

- *Guilt*—feeling guilty that I am somehow to blame for something I did or did not do for Mary, something that might have contributed in one way or another to her condition. I indulged in the "What if," "If I had only," "If I only knew" syndrome.

- *Sadness and Pity*—why did this happen to Mary? It isn't fair. How can I cope with this no-win situation? Nobody cares. I can't continue with this terrible problem. Is anyone out there listening?

- *Acceptance*—after all has failed to improve my wife's condition, there must be a grudging acceptance of the doctor's prognosis that Mary will not recover from her fatal illness. Finally I turned to God to help ease Mary's pain and suffering. This was a good time for the Serenity Prayer:

> "God grant me the serenity to accept the things I cannot change, the courage to change the things I can, and the wisdom to know the difference."

I often turned to God for help during extremely emotional situations. Sometimes there seemed to be a remote response through actions I took on hard problems which were solved with simple answers, which before the prayers seemed unsolvable. "Yes, Virginia, there is a God!"

In life education continues from birth to death. We learn something new every day. Caregiving became the learning experience of my life during these past years. Many lessons were learned during those long, hard, and lonely years, which, if I had known (there goes the big "If") them earlier, would have made my caregiving much easier, both mentally and physically.

I hope that the lessons I have learned and the information I have gathered will provide others with the knowledge and resources they need to prepare for their vitally important role in caring for a loved one. I hope to provide some clues on avoiding pitfalls, while giving you a basic understanding of what to expect down the road and perhaps help you eliminate some of the trial-and-error solutions other caregivers had to work through. I start with some of the organizations that helped me, for which I remain eternally grateful.

SUPPORT ORGANIZATIONS

Alzheimer's Association

I was in a completely exhausted condition when I first contacted the Honolulu chapter of the Alzheimer's Association. I learned a new word, *respite*. It means you can leave your loved one with them to get away for a few hours to do essential errands. This brief time apart provides a period of rest and relief for caregivers.

In early 1988 I was put on a waiting list. After continuous calls stretched out over several weeks, they finally called back to say I should bring Mary to the Shepperd's Center in downtown Honolulu on Mondays from 9 A.M. to 1 P.M. I was elated and eagerly looked forward to my first "respite relief."

I knew it would take me about forty-five minutes of driving time each way, and then there was the changing of Mary's diapers, packing her lunch and diaper bag, getting her into and out of the car, and so forth. Was it worth it just for a change of scenery for a few hours? The answer was a resounding yes, yes, yes!

Later I was authorized to bring Mary to another Alzheimer's respite location in Kalihi—giving me another four hours of free time on Wednesdays. I was overjoyed. That only gave me 160 hours per week to see to Mary's needs. This was a much-needed respite at a critical time for which I was very thankful.

The Alzheimer's chapter also sponsored *support group* meetings along with many meetings and seminars on caregiving and related matters. While in these groups I met some fine people who remain my close friends.

Like all good things the respite didn't last long. After a few months I received my first "Dear Frank" letter stating that Mary's condition needed a higher level of care. Due to her incontinence and other advancing problems they were unable to care for her at their respite locations. This was a serious blow, like the loss of your best friend. One step forward and two steps back!

State-Sponsored Health Program

I always checked out each facility or caregiver through interviews, checking references, the level of care given, reputation of the facility or person, and talking with others who have had their loved ones under their care. There are many ways to be safe rather than sorry.

My next attempt to locate help was the Hawaii state-sponsored program at the Windward Health Center in Kaneohe, near my home.

In mid-1989 public health nurse Karen Crozier was organizing a new program of day care for the elderly. She said it could offer Mary four hours of care on Wednesdays. After a slow start the facility was able to expand to include Mondays. What a help! This arrangement was good for several months. Then I received their version of a "Dear Frank" letter indicating Mary needed a higher level of care, so this respite was terminated. The culprit was incontinence.

The Windward Health Center also had a program called the "Senior Companion." This included a qualified senior citizen who was sent to your home to care for your patient for four hours during the day. Mary was cared for on Monday and Tuesday mornings during the last few months of her life. This is a good program.

Senior Day-Care Center

I did much research before finding the Windward Senior Day-Care Center in Kailua in 1990. After working through the waiting list routine I was able to bring Mary there on Fridays from 9 A.M. to 4:30 P.M. This was a real break for me. Later I was able to extend Mary's care to two days and finally to five days per week. This was my first real respite in many months. This arrangement lasted for several months, then came the dreaded "Dear Frank" notice stating the same problem. Mary needed a higher level of care. At this stage I really felt down. I didn't want to start over again.

My options were quickly narrowing since there were few facilities left: long-term care, which was very costly (approximately $45,000.00 annually—*if* you can get in); live-in care (in short supply); and part-time care (also in short supply).

Ann Pearl Intermediate Care Facility

The next stop for Mary was at the Ann Pearl Intermediate Care Facility in Kaneohe. Most patients were full-time residents. A few patients were selected for the small day-care program operating Mondays through Fridays from 8 A.M. to 5 P.M. In late 1991 I was able to get Mary in one day per week, and for a short time prior to her death she was accepted for two days. Here they fed her, gave required medication, changed her, and made her comfortable. It helped me a lot at this late stage of her disease.

I was extremely lucky to get her into this program. I had been on the waiting list for over a year. Here again, *patience* and *persistence* paid off. Mary remained in this program till her death.

Other Programs

In addition to the facilities discussed above, there are several other *private caregivers* who provide a wide range of care either in your home or theirs for an hourly rate. The price is high, but in some cases negotiable.

Trying to find a qualified and reliable caregiver is always a challenge. Good places to look for them include support organizations, hospital programs, city and state health departments, and talking to other caregivers and satisfied customers. After selecting one, conduct interviews, check references, and check with families who have hired them before.

Home Care Program

Another source to check is called *Home Care Program,* usually sponsored by several area hospitals. It is Medicare-covered for qualified patients, and care is given and supervised by a registered nurse. Nurse's aides and attendants perform most of the duties in your home.

Mary finally met the qualifications of the Castle Medical Center's home care program in Kailua during the last two months of her life. A nurse's aide would change, clean, and give Mary a bath (on the bed); wash her hair; and tend to any ongoing problems twice a week. They complete their work within two hours during each visit.

This is a very good program. The Medical Center program representative visited our home to evaluate Mary for need and me to see if I qualified to receive the assistance.

It's up to the caregiver to contact those who operate such programs; they do not solicit your business. Remember to exercise patience and be persistent during the execution of your caregiving functions.

A SUMMARY OF KEY LESSONS LEARNED

1. Never turn down any offer of help or assistance.

2. Aggressively seek assistance for your patient's needs as well as your own.

3. Learn as much as you can about the illness or condition affecting your loved one.

4. Learn as much as you can about the medication to be prescribed.

5. Research all facets of federal, state, and county assistance available to you and your patient.

6. The caregivers must maintain good mental and physical health.

7. Select the right doctor for the specific needs and problems of your patient.

8. Carefully screen caregivers who come into your home.

9. Seek and get assistance from your various family members.

10. Check all sources for respite for yourself.

11. Find, join, and participate in support groups established for your patient's disease.

12. Never blame the patient for his/her condition or actions.

13. Always prepare a "fact sheet" on your patient.

14. Obtain a durable power of attorney for your patient-spouse prior to the patient's incapacitation.

15. Review and update your family estate planning.

16. Be prepared for the death of your patient.

17. After the death, get on with the rest of your life.

1. Never turn down any offer of help or assistance.

Eagerly *accept* whatever is offered—material, physical, monetary, or moral support. As a novice in the field of caregiving early on, I felt I could easily handle this complex situation. I was sure I could formulate a plan, establish a routine, organize things, then execute the plan. The concept works well in the military or in business, but not so in the aggressive atmosphere of caregiving, where the landscape changes daily. In caregiving, something new and complicated often happens to a human body on a continuing "real-time" basis.

Accept the fact that you can't do it by yourself! You will need help! With help you can survive to give care. Without help you could become as much of a casualty as the patient.

2. Aggressively seek assistance for your patient's needs as well as your own.

There are plenty of people and facilities out there who *do care* and *will assist* you. However, you must take the initiative to seek out and select those who can be of help to you. For the first few months I took care of Mary, it wasn't just an eight-to-five job. It was round the clock—day and night. I was responsible. Even the strong and healthy will soon succumb to the pressure of trying to meet the diverse challenges of a debilitating illness.

3. Learn as much as you can about the illness or condition affecting your loved one.

Discuss matters in detail with the doctor. Understand the diagnosis and its implications for the near term and the long term. *Don't be afraid to ask questions.* Your doctor will be glad to respond. With the information you learn from the doctor, do some independent research at home, in medical books, and at the library. Courses and seminars are often available on caregiving of specific diseases. Federal, state, county, and city as well as local university and hospital health programs sponsor many of these functions.

Sometimes you can bring your loved one to the functions. The sponsors will provide care for the patient while you attend the class. This results in an added respite bonus for you.

When offered a chance to attend one of these courses or seminars, take it! You'll learn a lot about the illness, how to care for the person affected, and what to do in daily and emergency situations. These actions will better prepare you to care for your relative and for updating and discussing the person's status with the doctor.

4. Learn as much as you can about the medication to be prescribed.

Ask the doctor what the *prescribed medication* is supposed to do for the patient, whether there are any reactions to expect, any side effects to watch for, and any likely interactions with other prescribed medications your loved one is taking.

A number of guides to prescription drugs are published and readily available. Get a current copy to review details of the drugs involved so you may better understand and react when necessary. Copies are available at your local library.

5. Research all facets of federal, state, and county assistance available to you and your patient.

Be sure to check *Medicare* and *Medicaid* programs and your patient's eligibility. Local offices can easily determine if you qualify and provide you with proper procedures to receive aid.

Many state departments of health have programs for the aging and related services for senior citizens. They are worth checking out.

Caregivers who are retired from the *military,* or are caring for someone who is, should check with the local military authorities to determine what type of medical assistance they are qualified to receive, including doctor's visits, hospital coverage, and special pharmacy rates.

Don't forget to look into local hospital and university programs. They offer a wide range of assistance.

6. Caregivers must maintain good mental and physical health.

The person in need of care is totally dependent on you for his/her life. You must be able to perform your caregiver function. The job is a tough one that requires you to be alert and able to respond to all challenges. This requires excellent mental and physical health.

I have detailed care for the caregiver in chapter 11.

7. Select the right doctor for the specific needs and problems of your patient.

A *neurologist* is the suggested medical specialist for problems of the brain, and dementia in particular. Read up on your patient's problems, ask questions, and be sure to take a notebook to record information given by the doctor. Don't try to keep all the information in your head. Go slow and get it right. If you don't your loved one may be the one who suffers.

If you believe you have a good reason, don't hesitate to get a second opinion from another doctor.

Establishing a good relationship with your doctor is very important. This can be enhanced by doing your homework before you take your relative for a visit to the doctor. Asking lots of relevant questions and giving good patient update reports on actions and reactions means better care. Don't forget, you are with the patient on a daily basis and are in a position to witness the subtle symptoms and reactions of the patient. This is information the doctor doesn't have. Your accurate reporting will result in a better evaluation and treatment of the patient and an improved relationship with your doctor.

8. Carefully screen caregivers who come into your home.

Your home is your castle, and your valued possessions should not be put at risk. Very carefully screen all part-time or full-time applicants. Also consider the source who recommended the applicant to you. Are they reliable?

You can learn much through a face-to-face interview. To conduct a proper interview you must be prepared in advance. Prepare an outline and a series of questions, then follow the outline and be sure to get complete answers to your questions.

If you feel secure that you have the right person, then check references to confirm your impression. Talk with other patients' families who have used the person's services. What do they say about the applicant's performance? Also, verify the telephone and address of the potential caregiver for your relative. It's better to be *safe* than sorry.

9. Seek and get assistance from your various family members.

Your family has a responsibility to assist in caring for others within the family, particularly the mother and father. Seek any type of help they can give: monetary, physical, or possibly just moral support. Many times it will not be easy due to family situations, distances separating family members, and the circumstances of each person. To obtain such help it is necessary to share confidences of your ability to handle the care with your relatives. Sometimes pride prevents you from seeking help from others in the family. If you need help—*ask!*

10. Check all sources for respite for yourself.

The longer you perform caregiver functions the more you must depend on *respite*—that time away from caregiving that permits you to recharge and to be your own person. Actively seek out the programs that can help you. Most programs will accept you depending on availability, wait lists, and other factors. Don't give up. Be persistent and exercise patience.

Respite offers a safe and caring place where you can leave

your loved one for a specific time while you are free to do things you must do. As you progress in your tasks you will realize the importance of its benefits. It is rest and relief for the caregiver.

11. Find, join and participate in support groups established for your patient's disease.

Support groups are formed for almost all major medical problems, including dementia. Don't overlook this key part of your strategy for solving your care-related problems.

This is an outstanding means of venting your frustrations with people who have or are going through the same trauma as you. They become the teachers and you the student in learning how they coped or are coping and solving their problems. It is welcome news to know that you're not alone and that others understand. Others in the group may be experiencing the same or possibly worse problems.

An added bonus for you is the *camaraderie* you'll experience in meeting new people who are grappling with problems similar to yours and who speak your language.

12. Never blame the patient for his/her condition or actions.

Always remember that those who suffer from dementia and related diseases have no control over conditions or actions. Blaming and confronting them only complicates the situation and results in a more confused patient. Put yourself in their place. Be tender and loving in handling those in your care. They can sense abrasive or resentful actions on your part, which will only compound an already stressful situation for both of you. Love and tenderness will calm the patient and relax you as well.

In all your caregiving functions, if you use humor and have patience it will pay off tenfold—for both of you.

13. Always prepare a "fact sheet" on your patient.

Whenever you leave your loved one in the hands of another care-giver, a care home, or a day care facility, be sure to prepare a *fact sheet* to assist them in their care. The fact sheet should include the person's present condition; the specific care requirements, including medication, food supplements, clothes, and diapers; emergency instructions; and the name and telephone number of the person's doctor. Also include your itinerary and where you can be reached at all times during your absence.

I have included a copy of the last fact sheet I prepared for Mary (see pp. 125–28). It was given to the care home during her temporary stay there in July 1992. It includes a detailed briefing to the supervising nurse at the facility when I delivered Mary into their care. It contained specific instructions on preventing choking. I also gave them a suction machine as a precaution.

The caregiver should always brief the head nurse at the care facility on the fact sheet and other care requirements.

The same briefing should be given to any caregiver who comes into your home to care for your relative.

14. Obtain a durable power of attorney for your patient-spouse prior to the patient's incapacitation.

Caregivers of persons with progressive and degenerative dementia should be aware of several important legal actions. This is a must. If you do not have a *durable power of attorney,* begin the process of securing it while your family member is still capable of signing it. This document gives the caregiver legal power to sign for, sell, and invest any and all assets owned by your spouse or jointly owned by the two of you. In the event of the unexpected death of your patient you will be able to handle assets in his/her name. Without this important document you may have trouble in these areas.

The durable power of attorney also allows you control of these assets when the patient becomes incapacitated. You can act on his/her behalf in matters of medical and health situations as well. Without such legal authority established ahead of time major decisions may require a court order. Don't overlook this very important matter. When exercising a power of attorney your management of any assets involved can be audited.

A separate power of attorney can also be obtained to serve a specific purpose: for example, for health purposes or selling a car.

15. Review and update your family estate planning.

An in-depth *estate planning* must be done to look into all your financial wealth with a clear plan for disposal of that wealth upon your death or that of your patient (spouse). This planning is doubly important when your spouse has a disease as serious and debilitating as Mary's dementia.

After a review of all your assets, including your investment and real-estate portfolios, you will be able to determine what additional legal actions are necessary for your loved one. Several options are available, including a *Living Trust*. This document is a means of assigning wealth while the patient is still alive so that its distribution takes place at the time of death, eliminating the high cost of probating a will with its attendant high attorney costs. This should be checked out with a tax attorney or certified public accountant.

A *Living Will*, if appropriate, should be prepared for both you and your patient-spouse. This will give instructions to the doctor and hospital on how to respond to emergency conditions and the extent of life-saving techniques to use or not use on your loved one under such circumstances.

Sometimes *resuscitation orders* are discussed with physicians. This condensed version of the living will identifies the extent of life-saving techniques to apply to the patient during emergency or life-and-death situations. This document is also given to the doctor.

If applicable, a review of the *life insurance policies* should be conducted. Be sure you know where the policies are located, that the premiums are paid to date, and the provisions for death benefits are clearly understood.

The patient's *last will and testament* should be current and its location known. The document should clearly identify who is to carry out the provisions of the will.

Sooner or later all family caregivers are faced with one or more of these important matters. Be prepared so the shock of death and its emotional stress will not find you unprepared to make critical decisions after your loved one has died.

16. Be prepared for the death of your patient.

The death of the person you have cared for can be a highly *emotional* event. There are many actions you must take immediately thereafter. First, try to relax. If you aren't the person who has been designated to make all funeral arrangements for the deceased, then the individual with that responsibility should be notified immediately. If you will be the responsible party and have a plan of action, update it. If you don't, then prepare one now. The following should be included in your plan:

- Notify close relatives by telephone.

- Determine if organ donation is to be done. What are the deceased's wishes?

- Select a mortuary and method of delivering the body to that location.

- Select method of burial: interment or inurnment (cremation).

- Select the burial site and headstone, if appropriate.

- Select a casket or urn to hold the remains.

- Select the type of burial ceremony.

- Prepare the obituary.

- Prepare and send death notices. In Hawaii notification of death is normally prepared and sent by the mortuary to the State Department of Health and other appropriate authorities. I composed and sent personal death notices to all our relatives and close friends.

- Be aware that an autopsy may be required. In Hawaii, if the death is accidental, an autopsy is mandatory.

- Select the floral display for the burial site.

- Select those to attend the ceremony.

- Select the person to officiate.

- Prepare eulogies to be given.

- Arrange transportation of the body or urn to the burial site.

These are some of the essential points to address once the death has occurred.

17. After the death, get on with the rest of your life.

After the burial and an appropriate period of adjustment for the grief process, you need to consider your alternatives and get on with the rest of your life. If after this time has passed you still have difficulty with your loss, it might be time to consider counseling. The Alzheimer's Association or other organization should have information about *bereavement groups* and counseling services. Everyone needs time to work out their feelings. There is no right or wrong way to grieve. It is an individual and very personal process that fits the background, personality, and emotional makeup of the bereaved. If you need help in the process, it's available for you.

I urge you to disassociate yourself from self-pity. Your life is not over. There are *new horizons* for you to challenge. Seek them out and set new goals, then go out and meet those goals head-on.

Several additional areas included in lessons learned are shown in the following sequence.

1. A sample copy of a "fact sheet" I prepared for Mary and gave to the care home in July 1992, as discussed in lesson number 13.

2. A sample copy of a "fact sheet" for Mary given to caregivers coming into our home to care for Mary. This is distinct from the care home sheet shown earlier.

3. An outline of a typical day's care for Mary during noncrisis situations from being awakened in the morning to getting tucked into bed at night.

Finally, don't hesitate to use religion for spiritual support. Also carefully consider your budget limitations in determining the type and scope of needed care for your patient.

I have identified some of the compelling lessons I learned during my role as a caregiver and there are others I did not. I'm hopeful that these lessons will benefit other caregivers. *Good luck!*

SAMPLE COPY

FACT SHEET—MARY M. WALL

(as of July 1992)

DIAGNOSIS: Multi-infarct-dementia, Parkinson's disease, and possible Alzheimer's disease.

PRESENT CONDITION: Totally dependent for everything; totally incontinent (urine and bowel); unable to talk, stand, walk, dress, feed self, or sit on toilet. She needs assistance for everything.

PRIMARY DOCTOR: Dr. James F. Pierce—Neurologist—Phone _____
Dr. Ficke—Internal Medicine, Tripler—Phone_____
Dr. Palma—Internal Medicine, Kailua—Phone _____

MEDICATION: *Aspirin-Enteric pd* 325mg* (Ecotrin®): 1 tablet daily, given with applesauce before breakfast.

Ascorbic Acid pd 500mg: 2 tablets taken daily—halved during morning and evening meals.

Thiamine HCL pd 50 mg: 2 tablets taken daily—halved during morning and evening meals.

Estrogen conjugated pd .625mg: 1 tablet taken daily—first 25 days of each month—before breakfast with applesauce.

Calcium Carbonate pd 50mg: 1 tablet taken 3 times daily—halved during meals.

---

*pd stands for "prescribed dosage."

Lactulose pd 10gm/a5ml: 3 tablespoons taken with juice thickened with applesauce or Thick-It® before breakfast and dinner meals.

FOOD SUPPLEMENT: I give her one can of "TWO-CAL" daily (455 cal). I left one can for each day she will be at the care home. I am also leaving a thickener called Thick-It® for use in liquids.

INCONTINENCE: She is diapered 24 hours daily—both bladder and bowel. I use flat diapers with diaper pins to close gaps on legs.

EATING: Unable to feed self. She is on a low cholesterol-high fiber diet. All food must be processed to puree texture. She usually has problems getting started. If too much in mouth she will cough it up—choking and food aspiration is always a risk so feed her slowly and carefully.

DRINKING: She needs lots of liquid during the day. Usually a very slow process. She has a hard time swallowing liquid in morning; thicken the liquid with applesauce or Thick-It.®

GLASSES: Need cleaning daily and in between when necessary. Change nose pads when required.

TALKING: Unable to talk or have a conversation. Sometimes she seems to respond to soft music—with her eyes.

STIFFNESS: She is rigid with her right leg "contracted." Her hands are curling inward; for this I use a "holding pad" in each hand—this helps. She squeezes them.

WALKING: Unable to walk or stand unaided.

SHOWER: Needs one daily. If shower stool is used be careful it does not cause abrasion on tailbone.

DRESSING: Cannot dress or undress herself. It must be done for her. During day she uses diapers and dusters. At night uses nightgowns with a slit or open back. At night use double diapers.

GROOMING: She can't do it—needs your help. Loves to have hair combed and massage with electric massager—in neck and head areas.

TOILETING: She can't do it—no control over urine or BMs—diapered 24 hours daily.

FINGERNAILS: Need to be cut short—she gouges herself with long fingernails. Her toenails also need trimming. Has very strong grip.

SLEEPING: She sleeps on her back. Once in bed she usually goes to sleep and does not move until I get her up around 6:30 A.M. Try to get her to bed by 7 P.M. Put additional diaper on bed for insurance.

TEETH: She has upper and lower dentures. I soak them overnight—just before I put her to bed.

SWEATING: She sweats when diapers are full or when she has a fever. She has had urinary tract infections in the past.

TELEVISION: Sometimes she looks at it; I'm sure she doesn't follow. Likes music—oldies—classical—soft music.

SUMMARY: She needs help for everything.

CAUTION: BE CAREFUL not to give her food or liquids too fast or too thin or thick. ASPIRATION OF FOOD and CHOKING could result.

EMERGENCY: If hospitalization is required—take her to the emergency room at Tripler Army Medical Center. I have attached a copy of Mary's medical card. Present it at the ER desk.

EMERGENCY—Contact me (FRANK A. WALL) when I am off-island during 7–22 July 1992 at:

Dates	Telephone	Name	Location
7–9 July			Mt. View, Calif.
9–13 July			Baltimore, Md.
13–22 July			Virginia Beach, Va.

SOURCE: FRANK A. WALL—Husband and primary caregiver for wife.

SAMPLE COPY

MARY M. WALL—Home care

The following information is shown to assist caregivers who care for MARY at her home during the period 12:30–4:30 P.M.

- Give medication with applesauce 30 minutes prior to lunch as per instructions.

- Feed Mary lunch at approximately 1–1:15 P.M. Use microwave oven for heating. Process food to puree per verbal instructions.

- Give 2–3 glasses of water or juice, thicken with applesauce or Thick-It®. Spoon-feed slowly to prevent choking.

- Walk or stand Mary for at least 1 hour—as per instructions.

- Take for wheelchair ride each day, weather permitting, using route as discussed.

- When BM or urination occurs—change her in bedroom, use wipes and safety pins on diaper legs to prevent leaking. This is a good time to exercise her arms and legs—as per instructions.

- Clip her finger- and toenails—as required.

- Use electric massager—she loves this! Concentrate on head and base of spine. Also massage both hands daily.

- Shave legs—when required. Comb hair periodically.

- Place her in chair provided on lanai—weather permitting.

- Play selected music periodically—as per instructions.

- Apply Intensive Care® lotion to her face and arms daily.

- Check her for "wetness" just prior to leaving for the day and change if needed.

- CAUTION! Do not administer food or liquid too fast— choking could result.

- Other: Perform light housekeeping tasks as directed.

A TYPICAL DAY'S CARE

Caring for Mary was a multifaceted task. This was a typical day's schedule from wake-up in the morning to being tucked into bed for the night.

Morning

Rise about 6:30 A.M. Get diapers and accessories ready, select Mary's clothes for the day, and bring wheelchair into bedroom for transport.

Check Mary. Remove her soiled diapers and nightgown and place them in specially prepared receptacles. Inspect her skin around the pubic area for irritation and wash her with a soft cloth to ensure that all urine has been removed.

Apply medication (Lotrimin®) to skin, if appropriate. Also lightly powder in front and back.

Lay diaper under Mary, using a body-rolling method. Secure clean diaper with a large safety pin on each leg to prevent potential leaks.

Dress Mary with selected dress. I always used dusters (house-dresses) with snaps down the front for ease in dressing.

Many times after completing all of the above, Mary would release a large volume of urine. Then all these steps would be repeated.

Lift Mary out of bed and place her into the wheelchair for transport to her seat in the family room.

The next step is to give her orange juice, but she is unable to swallow it so I add a Thick-It® product to thicken the liquid and spoon-feed it to her until the glass is empty.

I play a tape of her favorite classical music, while I go for a walk, swim in the pool, or do other exercise. (This was only possible during the latter stages of her illness when she was unable to move.)

Breakfast

I then prepare Mary's morning meal, consisting of hot oatmeal, unprocessed bran, fruit (applesauce, peaches, pears, pineapple, or other fresh fruit), skim milk, and a slice of whole wheat bread all processed into a puree texture, and spoon-feed to Mary.

I follow this with a glass of the food supplement Ensure Plus®, using Thick-It® which is also spoon-fed.

This menu varies during the week.

Showering

After breakfast I check her diaper, which is usually wet or full. We then wheel into the bedroom to prepare her for her daily shower. I transport Mary into the bathroom, lift her into the *shower chair* positioned in the shower, and proceed to clean, rinse, and dry her. Then we return to the bedroom to check her skin thoroughly for irritation or other problems. If necessary I treat problem skin areas and place new diapers on, dress her, and transport Mary back to her seat in the family room.

I then give her a glass of juice, water, or other liquid.

Day Care

One of three actions then takes place.

1. If I take Mary to a day-care facility, I check her diaper again, change her if necessary, pack her diaper bag and her required medication, and transport her to the car. Getting her there is always an interesting experience, but I find new ways to simplify it. (Several times after she was settled in the car and we were ready to go, I noticed a terrible odor of urine or BM. This required me to return to the bedroom to change her and repeat all these procedures.) We arrive at the day-care facility and I give Mary's medication and instructions for care to the appropriate caregiver.

2. If a temporary caregiver is scheduled to come into our home to care for Mary, I get her groomed and ready, prepare lunch for the caregiver to feed Mary, brief the caregiver on Mary's present condition, provide special instructions, and identify medication needed during care period.

3. If I am caring for Mary, I check her periodically and change her when necessary. If weather permits I take her for a wheelchair ride over a designated route, play music, perform personal care such as nails, combing hair, exercising her arms and legs, administering her medications, read to her, and give liquids.

Lunch

While at home I prepare and feed Mary her lunch about 12:15. Lunch consists of soup, chicken, vegetables, and bread, all of which are pureed and spoon-fed. I also give her required medication and other liquids. She is always changed and cleaned prior to feeding.

(In the later stages of her disease Mary continually had eating problems, primarily involving swallowing and coughing. Aspiration of food into the lungs was a constant serious threat, and as a result, feeding took a long time to complete.)

Visits to Doctors

Visits to doctors, clinics, hospitals, pharmacies, and laboratories seem continuous. X rays for aspiration and various infections, lab tests for urinary infections, new and follow-up appointments, update briefings to doctors on Mary's status, and trying to solve old problems and deal with new ones are all phased into daily schedules, including unscheduled visits to the hospital emergency room during crisis situations. Time goes by very quickly with all this activity. Before I realize it I'm facing dinner.

If Mary is at a day-care facility I pick her up and transport her into the car, then back to our house. She is usually wet and in need of changing. Upon arrival at home, I change her diaper and check her for irritation. Sometimes she needs immediate treatment. I also change her dress and clean her so she's ready for dinner. She looks drained and very tired when I pick her up at the care home. She seems much more relaxed after I freshen her up a bit, giving her liquids and some tender loving care.

Dinner

We eat dinner around 6:30. Before doing so I take time to change Mary again, give her medication, and treat her infections, if any. I play some classical or "oldie" music while I prepare the evening meal at about 5:00.

Dinner for Mary consists of a salad (lettuce, tomatoes, celery, carrots, broccoli, etc.), chicken, fish, or lean meat with no fat, baked potatoes, vegetables (corn, string beans, onions, or other fresh vegetables), a piece of whole wheat bread and unprocessed bran. The salad and main course are processed to puree and spoon-fed separately. For dessert I puree fruits and ice cream with home-made cookies. After the meal it is finally time to relax (?) prior to getting Mary ready for night.

Preparing Mary for Bed

At approximately 8:15 I wheel Mary from the family room to her bedroom for night processing.

I lay her on the bed, remove her soiled diapers and dress, inspect her, and clean and treat any infections or irritations. Before putting Mary to bed I always place a waterproof sheet and a flat diaper on the bed under Mary. This protects the bed from any urine or BM leakage. Then I place a large diaper around her and secure it on her legs with a large safety pin to prevent leaking.

Next, I use a nightgown with a *slit* in the back for ease in dressing her. When I'm ready I transport her to the bed and tuck her in for the night. Amen!

(In the later stages of her disease she would not normally move or turn. However, in the early stages she was very active. I could never leave her alone anywhere. This resulted in use of a posey restraint to prevent her from falling out of her bed, her chair, or the wheelchair.)

15

Medical Aids

In carrying out the responsibilities of the caregiver, it is necessary to obtain certain *medical aids* to assist the patient and the caregiver in everyday living. I will discuss some of the aids I used in caring for Mary.

Adult diapers. These were used primarily for urine incontinence to prevent soiling everything she was wearing, sat on, or slept on. Later they were used for bowel incontinence as well.

Dentures. Mary's dentures proved to be an extremely valuable asset in performing dental hygiene. The ease in inserting and extracting them for cleaning was simple compared to the struggle to clean a normal set of teeth in such a patient. If your patient has dentures, be thankful. It saves much extra work.

Doughnut cushion. An air-inflated cushion which looks like a small swimming tube. It is used for the patient to sit on when in one place for an extended time period and/or for an ulcerous condition.

Duoderm pads. A specially processed bandage used to protect and heal bedsores and ulcers on your patient. Once the condition is identified, treated, and cleaned, the pads are applied and remain on the ulcer or sore for several days before changing. They are very effective.

Dusters. This is a housecoat with an open front using snaps to close. Its use enables the caregiver to simplify dressing, undressing, and changing diapers. Mary's nightwear as well as daywear was restricted to clothing which did not have pullover features. Nightwear clothing was slit in the back, with ties for ease in preparing the patient for bed.

Eggshell pillow. Provides a better and more comfortable surface for the head and neck. It conforms to the contours of the patient.

Food processor. Although this is food-oriented it is a medical necessity to prepare pureed textured food for patients who cannot swallow whole food. This was vital to Mary's survival. Many meals and desserts tailored to her needs were routinely processed on this device. I still use it daily.

Grab bars. These are a must for use in shower and toilet locations. They are safety devices and can prevent serious injury to your patient. Install them before you need them. I still use the one in my shower on a daily basis, depending on it as a security item.

Handgrips. Mary's hands started *curling* inward with fingernails digging into her flesh on the hands. To counter this I used a rolled and covered wool sock as a handgrip for each hand. Use of this handgrip along with keeping her fingernails trimmed short helped ease the intensity of the curling and prevented her from digging into her flesh.

Handheld shower head. Used in conjunction with the shower chair to wash and clean the patient.

Hospital bed. Used for bedridden patients or for those who must be secured at night with guard rails.

Humor and laughter. I noticed when humor and laughter were used, it seemed to pacify or bring out signs of smiling and acceptance of these emotions.

Love. The most *important ingredient* of caregiving. All your actions for the patient should be tender and caring, not abrasive or resentful or from self-motivated thoughts. Showing love to your patient has a healing and soothing effect on the loved one. Sometimes this is hard to do under the stressful situations you will encounter. If you try it you will also be helped.

Music. It has a profound *therapeutic* effect on the patient. It soothes and calms the patient, particularly those tapes or records dating back to the patient's youthful years. Mary loved music and I believe she looked forward to the daily music played for her. It also was helpful for the caregiver.

Patience. A *must* for the caregiver. Getting mad at the patient will be counterproductive and only compounds the problem, while the patience approach will result in a more soothing atmosphere for both the patient and the caregiver.

Plastic mattress cover. Prevents urine and other leaks from getting into the mattress. It saves a lot of extra work.

Plastic pillow cover. Protects the pillow from sweat and other means of soiling.

Portable suction machine. Used to prevent choking while being fed. It is a device similar to the dentist's suction machine. The patient's throat can be cleared of phlegm or other mucus by using this machine. This was used in the later stages of Mary's disease progression. It can be obtained from most medical supply centers. *Use this device only under doctor's guidance.*

Posey restraint. A device to *secure* the patient that is put on the patient like a sweater. It has tie strings which attach to the patient's seat, wheelchair, or bed to prevent falling. This device was used almost daily during the early stages of Mary's illness. Later it was unnecessary since Mary's movement declined rapidly during the final stages.

Shower chair. For use when the patient is unable to stand in the shower. The patient can be seated while being showered and then be lifted into and out of the shower chair into the waiting wheelchair.

Small sliding bolt for entrance doors. To be installed near the top and bottom of doors. To keep the "wandering" patient in the house or to prevent from straying into unsafe areas.

Thick-It®. A product used to thicken liquids given to patients having trouble swallowing liquids or solids. It helps to prevent choking and aspiration of food into the lungs.

Waffle mattress. Used for the patient who must sit or lie on the bed for long periods. It provides a more comfortable surface, particularly if the patient has bedsores or ulcers. It is also called an eggshell mattress.

Wheelchair. Used as a primary means of movement of the patient from one location to another. Use of this device became an indispensable item in caring for Mary. Be sure to select the right wheelchair for your patient. I found the wheelchair with small wheels in front and back was the one that fit Mary's needs since she was unable to coordinate the hand-propelling function using the type with large back wheels. It was much easier folding and placing it in the car or other storage areas. Consider use of a posey restraint to secure your patient in the wheelchair, if appropriate. I used the wheelchair inside and outside, when I would take Mary for rides in the open air. She liked these fresh air outings.

Evaluate your patient's needs for medical aids, procure them, and use them. As you progress in your caregiving activities you will find new and innovative ways to make things simpler. Be sure to keep an open mind in this area.

Although all of the items I discussed are not medical aids in the sense of hardware, they are in fact essential to the task of caregiving. A generous daily dose of *humor* and *laughter, love, and patience* will reap many rewards for you and the one you are caring for.

There are many potential areas of assistance in procuring the hardware items. Some of these may be procured through Medicare or Medicaid: if qualified, the military, if active or retired; or from commercial sources. Also check federal, state, city, county, hospital, university, and church programs and sources.

Help is out there but you must find the source to fit your specific needs.

16

Conclusion

After my seven years of caring for Mary, the only plausible answer I can give to the nagging question "Where did Mary go?" is that she now resides in a better place—free of pain and illness. In my heart, she will walk and talk, laugh and sing, for as long as I live.

The researchers, scientists, doctors, nurses, technicians, caregivers, and others concerned could not give positive medical identification of the state of Mary's mind, her fears, her thoughts, her pain threshold, what she could or could not understand, or her ability to cope or deal with her anxieties—all of which was brought on by the deadly progression of her illness.

Researchers are making slow progress in trying to identify the underlying causes of dementia so that preventive treatment can be developed to eradicate this incurable disease. Dementia affects millions of people across the country as it rapidly works its way through our nation's elderly population.

For many years dementia was believed to be a disease of senility or old age and nothing could be done about it. But researchers have found ways to slow down its effects. This progressive, dementing, and fatal brain disease is the fourth leading cause of death among U.S. adults. Yet efforts to secure needed funding for vital research for a cure are far behind the organized fundraising for the first three killers of our citizens: heart attack, cancer, and stroke.

Mary's case was more devastating than most since she was unfortunate to be afflicted with a combination of the worst kinds of dementia (the small strokes coupled with Alzheimer's disease) and aggravated by Parkinson's. After her loss of speech I was able to communicate with her for a limited time through touching her hands and eye communications; but after that, nothing.

In reality, two Marys were created: the original caring wife and mother and the second cloned through uncertainty, pain, confusion, indignity, fear, and the final complete deterioration of her mind and body. I am thankful that her suffering has ended and that she is now at peace.

Mary's death concluded my task as a caregiver, but I hope this book and the experiences conveyed in it—both Mary's and mine—will serve to inform and guide those who have yet to walk this physically demanding and emotionally rough path of caregiver for those innocent men and women who face the dark future of dementia.

Appendix

Glossary of Terms Associated with Dementia and Its Care

———◦•◦———

The medical profession, like all professions, has a unique *vocabulary* of its own. You must be familiar with this vocabulary so that you can better understand the range, scope, and care of your patient's disease.

This knowledge will materially assist you in following the discussion with doctors, nurses, technicians, and other medical providers about your patient's disease and the instructions for treatment, medication, and care. This will also provide a base for your understanding, particularly when the medical provider's use of unknown medical and technical terms is delivered at a rapid pace when your mind is at an emotional high and not receptive to learning new and complicated terms and procedures under stress conditions.

As you progress in your role of caregiver you will be exposed to many new medical terms. Write them down and look them up in a medical dictionary or vocabulary, which are available at your local library.

143

I have listed some of the terms I had to wrestle with during my many years of caregiving. Your early understanding of them will ease your burden.

Adult Day Care. A supervised program of medical and social services provided on an out-patient basis for those who qualify.

Alzheimer's Disease. An abnormal degeneration of the brain that causes loss of memory commonly associated with senility in the elderly. The disease progresses slowly, but within a few years the patient becomes bedridden and helpless. The cause is not known and there is no treatment.

Case Management. Client assessment of the patient, including identification and coordination of community resources upon qualification.

Catheter. A tube inserted into the body cavity to extract or inject fluids.

Cat Scan. A machine that passes X rays through the patient's body from various angles, which enables a computer to build up three-dimensional images to pinpoint problems.

Decubitus Ulcer. The medical term for *bedsores*. Occurs in patients who are bedridden or unable to move. Mary had them at the base of her spine and on the sides of her hips.

Dementia. A disease that kills parts of the brain that control various mental and physical control mechanisms.

Digital Procedure. A procedure for removal of fecal products (bowel movements) from a bowel-impacted patient, by using a gloved hand and lubricated finger entering the anal tract and digging out the fecal products.

Durable Power of Attorney. A legal document which authorizes the person named in the document to act for the patient in all matters of managing and controlling the patient's assets, even if the patient becomes incapacitated.

Fecal Products. Products from bowel movements.

Festination Walk. A sensation of walking fast and falling forward at the same time.

Home-Delivered Meals. Meals delivered to the home of those who are unable to shop or prepare their own meals. Usually this is a state-, county-, or community-sponsored program.

Hospice Services. Medical, nursing, and social services to provide support and reduce suffering for the dying and their families.

Identification Bracelet. Used to identify the mentally impaired, confused, or wandering patient. The patient's name, telephone number, and the disease are etched on the inside of the bracelet and worn by the patient. This is a very important item for those who are ambulatory. It is also called *Medic Alert.* Contact the local Alzheimer's Association for a free bracelet.

Incontinence. An involuntary release of urine (bladder) and bowel movement products.

Living Will. A legal document which spells out the degree of life-saving techniques to be used or not to be used in a life-threatening situation. Copies are to be given to your doctor or care facility.

Medicaid. A federal health program, similar to Medicare, administered by the state for qualified residents.

Medicare. A federal health program for those who meet the qualifications, which provides medical, hospital, medication, and other services and benefits.

MRI Scan. A Magnetic Resonance Imagery procedure using a laser-scanning device to determine ongoing status in the patient's brain or other body parts.

Multi-Infarct-Dementia. Repeated *strokes* that destroy small areas of the brain. The cumulative effect of this damage leads to dementia. Multi-infarct-dementia affects the memory, coordination, speech, or all of these functions, depending on the areas of the brain damaged. In Mary's case further minor strokes occurred and the progression of the disease could not be stopped.

Night Lights. A low-wattage light used in bedrooms and bathrooms at night to help prevent falling or accidents in the dark.

Nose Tube. A tube inserted through the nostril and into the patient's stomach as a means of providing nourishment and liquid feeding.

Nursing Home. Long-term full-care facility with doctor and registered nurse supervision.

Parkinson's Disease. A chronic disorder of the nervous system characterized by tremors, slow movements, and generalized body stiffness. This disease does not affect mental faculties, but they may appear to be impaired if the patient's speech is affected. There is no cure, but the symptoms can be controlled by medication. Mary used a medication called Sinemet® which was very effective in the early stages of the disease, but which became ineffective in time.

Patient's Fact Sheet. A detailed statement showing the present mental and physical condition of your patient, identifying required care and medication and where you can be reached at all times during your absence. Given to caregivers or care home charge nurses or others who are caring for your patient on a temporary basis.

Physical Therapy. Rehabilitative treatment for doctor-referred patients, provided by a skilled physical therapist.

Respite. A period of time of *rest and relief* for the caregiver away from the patient. Often it is a place to take the patient for care while the caregiver is free for other things.

Resuscitation Orders. Instructions to the doctor given by the patient's spouse or authorized representative, identifying the scope of life-saving techniques and procedures to be used or not to be used in life-threatening situations.

Short-Term Deficit. Inability to recall information the patient was exposed to after approximately 15 to 30 seconds. The memory then disappears and he/she must ask or look it up again.

Skilled Nursing Facility. A medically oriented full-time care facility administered by registered nurses.

Smoke Alarms. An alarm that should be installed at various locations where the patient resides.

Speech Therapy. Treatment for doctor-referred patients to help restore or improve speech of the patient, provided by skilled speech therapists.

Stomach Tube. A tube inserted into the patient's stomach to introduce nutrition (food, water, other liquids, and medication) when other means of feeding have failed. This tube is surgically inserted as a permanent means of feeding.

Syringe. An instrument for injecting fluids into the body or washing out body cavities or wounds.